D0274273

③ KSPA
WQ 18

DRCOG
Practice Exams:
MCQs, OSCEs and
Case Histories

Second edition

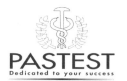

PASTEST
Dedicated to your success

DRCOG Practice Exams: MCQs, OSCEs and Case Histories
Second edition

Michael Dooley MMs FRCOG
Examiner for the Royal College of Obstetricians and Gynaecologists
Consultant Obstetrician and Gynaecologist
Dorset County Hospital, Dorchester, Dorset

Ali Elfara MD Dip(Obs) MRCOG
Specialist Registrar in Obstetrics and Gynaecology
Obstetrics and Gynaecology Department
Dorset County Hospital, Dorchester, Dorset

Michael Savvas FRCOG
Examiner for the Royal College of Obstetrics and Gynaecology
Consultant Obstetrician and Gynaecologist
King's College Hospital, London

First edition

Michael D. Read MD FRCSEd FRCOG
Examiner for the Royal College of Obstetricians and Gynaecologists
Consultant Obstetrician and Gynaecologist
Gloucestershire Royal Hospital, Gloucester

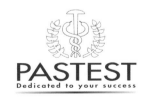

PASTEST
Dedicated to your success

© 2004 PASTEST LTD
Knutsford
Cheshire
Telephone: 01565 752000

All rights reserved. No part of this publication may be reproduced, stored in a retrieval system, or transmitted, in any form or by any means, electronic, mechanical, photocopying, recording or otherwise without the prior permission of the copyright owner.

First edition 1997
Second edition 2004

ISBN: 1 901198 96 0

A catalogue record for this book is available from the British Library.

The information contained within this book was obtained by PasTest from reliable sources. However, while every effort has been made to ensure its accuracy, no responsibility for loss, damage or injury occasioned to any person acting or refraining from action as a result of information contained herein can be accepted by the publishers or authors.

PasTest Revision Books and Intensive Courses
PasTest has been established in the field of postgraduate medical education since 1972, providing revision books and intensive study courses for doctors preparing for their professional examinations. Books and courses are available for the following specialties:
MRCP Part 1 and Part 2, MRCPCH Part 1 and Part 2, MRCS, MRCOG, MRCGP, DRCOG, MRCPsych, DCH, FRCA and PLAB.
For further details contact:
PasTest, Knutsford, Cheshire WA16 8DX
Tel: 01565 752000   Fax: 01565 650264
E-mail: enquiries@pastest.co.uk
Web site: www.pastest.co.uk

Typeset by Saxon Graphics Ltd, Derby
Printed by MPG Books Ltd, Bodmin, Cornwall

Contents

Introduction

This book is designed for candidates preparing to take the Diploma for the Royal College of Obstetricians and Gynaecologists. By kind permission of the Royal College of Obstetricians and Gynaecologists we have reproduced the information on the examination that the College routinely supplies to candidates. The lists of topics with which candidates are expected to be familiar are especially helpful, and these are backed up with a specific Revision Checklist prepared by a team of PasTest revision course lecturers.

There is no substitute for intensive revision based on MCQs that closely reflect the content and level of difficulty of the examination. This book contains three complete Practice Examinations each of 60 questions (five parts to each question) which can be taken under timed conditions to give candidates an accurate picture of the standard they have reached, and the topics which merit further revision. Correct answers and detailed explanatory notes are provided for every question.

October 1994 saw the introduction of the Objective Structured Clinical Examination (OSCE) as a means of assessment. This book includes 40 sample OSCE stations and 10 interactive case history stations together with practice questions which accurately reflect the type of material likely to be faced by candidates. Helpful advice on how to prepare for an examination of this type is also included. In the 'real' examination, every question is subjected to a rigorous committee assessment.

We hope that by using this book and taking part in PasTest's Intensive Revision Course for the DRCOG, candidates will cover most of the DRCOG syllabus as well as improve their standards of clinical care overall.

We would like to thank all those at PasTest for their patience and support, we would particularly like to thank Kirsten Baxter for her patient guidance and total professionalism.

Michael Dooley
Ali Elfara
Michael Savvas

Royal College Examination Regulations

Diploma examination regulations

The College awards a Diploma to fully registered medical practitioners who have had appropriate postgraduate training and who satisfy its examiners. The Diploma is intended to recognise a general practitioner's interest in obstetrics and gynaecology and is not a specialist qualification.

a. Candidates for the Diploma examination must be entered as fully registered medical practitioners in the Register of Medical Practitioners maintained by the General Medical Council or by the Medical Council of Ireland. The date of entry should be given and a copy of the current certificate of registration should be submitted.

b. The latest date for receiving the applications form is 1 February for the April examination or 1 August for the October examination.

   Candidates must submit a copy of their certificate of full registration with the completed application.

   Candidates must confirm that they are not currently suspended or removed from medical practice by any authorising body or involved in disciplinary proceedings related to medical practice in any country.

   The entry fee is payable in sterling at the time of application.

c. Candidates must complete a recognised combined appointment for six consecutive months. It is not essential to complete this training by the time of the examination. However, successful candidates will be required to provide a certificate confirming the completion of six months recognised training at the time of applying for registration as a Diplomate of the College.

   In special circumstances part-time clinical training in recognised posts is permitted provided approval of the College **is obtained in advance**.

   The training posts for the Diploma examination must be held in the United Kingdom or Republic of Ireland.

d. Council may refuse to allow a candidate to attempt the Diploma examination or become a Diplomate of the College. Under such circumstances the candidate will be advised of the appeals procedure.

e. No candidate may attempt the Diploma examination more than five times.

f. Candidates who withdraw their applications for a particular Diploma examination after the closing date or who fail to appear shall forfeit their examination fee.

g. Candidates must provide evidence of identification, **which includes name and photograph**, for inspection prior to commencement of the examination. Candidates failing to provide satisfactory evidence will not be allowed to attend the examination.

h. Successful candidates are required to pay a registration fee and, at the same time, provide a certificate confirming the completion of six months recognised training before being granted the Diploma of the Royal College of Obstetricians and Gynaecologists. The amount of the current registration fee is available from the Examination Secretary.

i. By applying to sit the DRCOG examination the candidate agrees to all the terms of the Diploma Examination Regulations and to the transfer of all copyright subsisting in examination material produced by the candidate to the College.

Cheques should be made payable to 'The Royal College of Obstetricians and Gynaecologists'. **Do not send cash.**

The Diploma examination

The examination will comprise:

(a) A multiple choice question (MCQ) paper lasting two hours examining areas of obstetrics, gynaecology and associated subjects. The paper will comprise of 60 five-part questions.

(b) An objective structured clinical examination (OSCE). This part of the examination may cover obstetrics, gynaecology, family planning, neonatology, or related subjects. There are 22 stations, each of six minutes, through which candidates rotate. Two of the stations are rest stations; at each of the other stations a task will be performed which may include a test of factual knowledge, problem solving, diagnosis, investigation and treatment and communication skills.

Question papers, answer sheets and examination materials remain the property of the College at all times.

Appeals against examination results

Written notification of intention to appeal must reach the College Secretary within 21 days from the date of issue of the result.

The Examination Committee has agreed the following guidelines for candidates and examiners regarding the DRCOG Examination.

Candidates should:

a. Appreciate the preventive role, and understand the significance of all routine procedures used in modern antenatal care.

b. Have an understanding of the epidemiology of maternal and perinatal morbidity and mortality as well as ethnic variations.

c. Be able to discuss the management of complications and life-threatening emergencies in early pregnancy.

d. Appreciate when those pregnant women initially suitable for shared care or full care by the general practitioner require referral for specialist opinion or care.

e. Understand the principles for pre-pregnancy evaluation and counselling of women faced with possible or real problems of fetal malformation.

f. Know the methods by which congenital malformation of the fetus may be detected.

g. Be aware of the methods of, and provision for, education in pregnancy, childbirth and the care of the newborn.

h. Understand the importance of social and emotional factors in pregnancy and childbirth.

i. Be able to understand and appreciate the risks of all types of antenatal and intrapartum infection for the mother, fetus and newborn infant.

j. Understand the role of the general practitioner, the midwife and that of the different members of the health-care team in care of pregnant women.

k. Understand the management of common conditions for which pregnant women are admitted to hospital, eg premature labour, pre-eclampsia, multiple pregnancy, fetal growth retardation, antepartum haemorrhage and maternal diseases.

l. Be able to recognise the symptoms and signs of the onset of labour.

m. Understand the principles, mechanisms and methods of management of normal and abnormal labour.

n. Understand the principles and methods which are used for the relief of pain in labour.

o. Understand the importance of accurate and detailed records in all aspects of obstetric care and recognise the value of such records in clinical audit.

p. Be able to carry out and discuss the routine examination of a newborn infant.

q. Understand and discuss the normal development of the newborn infant.

r. Recognise common diseases arising in the newborn infant.

s. Recognise congenital abnormalities in the newborn infant.

t. Understand how breast-feeding is established and maintained.

u. Recognise and treat all sources of infection in the puerperium.

v. Recognise and understand the management of physical and psychological problems of the mother in the postnatal period, eg puerperal depression.

w. Understand the normal involutional processes in the postpartum period.

x. Understand the indications for maternal immunisation with anti-D and rubella vaccine and the importance of confirming their efficacy.

And with regard to INTRANATAL CARE:

a. Understand the indications for the induction of labour.

b. Understand the physiology of uterine activity and the use of oxytocic drugs to augment uterine action.

c. Know the principles and practice of continuous fetal heart rate monitoring and acid–base studies.

d. Recognise and discuss the abnormalities that may occur in labour, eg fetal distress, haemorrhage, delay in labour, abnormal presentation, etc.

e.   be able to:
   (a)   Induce labour where appropriate.
   (b)   Provide obstetric analgesia and local anaesthesia, including pudendal block.
   (c)   Carry out a low forceps delivery and repair of the perineum.
   (d)   Resuscitate a shocked mother.
   (e)   Resuscitate a newborn baby.

a.   Understand the management of other abnormalities of labour, eg breech, twins, shoulder dystocia.

b.   Be able to manage the third stage of labour, including the management of postpartum haemorrhage and retained placenta.

c.   Be able to discuss the management of episiotomies and lacerations.

d.   Be aware of special arrangements needed for home confinements.

e.   Be able to communicate with women in labour so that they understand the procedures proposed for their own safety and that of their babies.

With regard to GYNAECOLOGY and GENITO-URINARY MEDICINE:

a.   Understand the role of the general practitioner in health education and preventive measures with regard to gynaecological diseases.

b.   Be able to take a gynaecological history, carry out a full and appropriate examination and conduct relevant investigations on patients of all ages.

c.   Understand the physical disorders due to congenital abnormalities of the female genital tract.

d.   Understand the principles involved in counselling patients with psychosexual problems.

e.   Be able to advise, investigate and manage patients complaining of infertility.

f.   Be able to manage all types of abortions in general practice, including diagnosis, emergency treatment and after-care.

g.   Understand the management of common menstrual disorders and the steps required to diagnose benign lesions of the genital tract and the principles regarding their management.

h.   Know the steps required for the detection of premalignant lesion of the cervix, the diagnosis of invasive neoplasia of the genital tract, and the general practitioner's role in the management of terminal cancer.

i.   Understand the physiology and management of the menopause.

j.   Understand the diagnosis and management of urinary tract disorders and of genital prolapse.

k.   Understand the diagnosis and management of patients suffering from vaginal discharges, infections of the genital tract and common vulval lesions.

l.   Understand sexually transmitted diseases and their treatment and control.

Family planning

It is expected that all candidates will have the same theoretical knowledge that is required by doctors who wish to take the Diploma of the Faculty of Family Planning and Reproductive Health Care of the RCOG, namely knowledge of:

a.   Acceptability of contraception.

b.   Choice of method and discussion of risks and benefits.

c.   All available contraceptive methods; necessary technical skills and management of associated complications including resuscitation.

d.   Male and female sterilisation.

e.   Abortion; counselling, legal aspects, techniques.

f.   Sexually transmitted diseases.

g.   Family planning services; organisation and administration (community, general practice, domiciliary and hospital).

h.   Well woman care.

'IT WILL THEREFORE BE APPROPRIATE FOR ANY ASPECT RELATED TO THESE DEFINED OBJECTIVES TO BE COVERED IN THE VARIOUS PARTS OF THE EXAMINATION, BUT IT DOES NOT PRECLUDE EXAMINERS FROM DISCUSSING OTHER TOPICS WHICH ARE RELEVANT TO GENERAL PRACTICE.'

DRCOG Revision Checklist

Preparation for the DRCOG examination can follow a structured approach using guidelines offered by the College at the time of application. The following is offered as a checklist that you can tick as you complete your revision in each area.

Obstetrics

History taking
- [ ] Examination of abdomen in pregnancy
- [ ] Perinatal mortality figures and causes
- [ ] Maternal mortality figures and causes
- [ ] Preconception evaluation and counselling

The diagnosis of pregnancy
- [ ] Antenatal care
- [ ] Role of the GP/Midwife/Primary health-care team Booking routines
- [ ] Criteria for GP care versus hospital care

Prenatal screening and diagnosis of abnormal α-fetoprotein
- [ ] Triple hormone assay
- [ ] Amniocentesis
- [ ] Ultrasound
- [ ] Chorionic villus biopsy

Common problems in pregnancy
- [ ] Placental insufficiency
- [ ] Intrauterine growth retardation
- [ ] Pre-eclampsia and hypertensive disease
- [ ] Diabetes and pregnancy
- [ ] Thyroid problems in pregnancy
- [ ] Anaemia
- [ ] Urinary tract infections
- [ ] Abdominal pain in pregnancy
- [ ] Heart disease
- [ ] Rhesus disease

- ☐ Antepartum haemorrhage
- ☐ Hydatidiform mole
- ☐ Hyperemesis
- ☐ Multiple pregnancy
- ☐ Hydramnios
- ☐ Fetal infection in pregnancy
- ☐ Preterm labour
- ☐ Premature rupture of membranes
- ☐ Prolonged pregnancy and post-maturity
- ☐ Intrapartum care
- ☐ Home deliveries versus hospital deliveries
- ☐ Fetal assessment
  - ☐ a. Doppler
  - ☐ b. Ultrasound
  - ☐ c. Cardiotocography
  - ☐ d. Kick chart
- ☐ Disseminated intravascular coagulation
- ☐ HELLP (haemolysis, elevated liver enzymes and a low platelet count) syndrome

Malpresentations

- ☐ Breech
- ☐ Unstable lie
- ☐ Transverse lie

Diagnosis of labour

- ☐ Physiology, mechanisms and management of normal labour
- ☐ Documentation/partograms
- ☐ Induction of labour criteria/methods
- ☐ Bishop's score

First stage

- ☐ Intrapartum monitoring
  - ☐ Cardiotocography
  - ☐ Scalp pH
- ☐ Intrapartum haemorrhage
- ☐ Pain relief
  - ☐ Epidural analgesia
  - ☐ Delay and management
  - ☐ Spinal analgesia

Second stage

- ☐ Definition
- ☐ Delay and management

- [ ] Instrumental deliveries
- [ ] Assisted breech delivery
- [ ] Concept of fetal distress
- [ ] Episiotomy and lacerations
- [ ] Caesarean section
- [ ] Shoulder dystocia
- [ ] Twin delivery

Third stage

- [ ] Active management
- [ ] Concept of oxytocin (syntometrine)
- [ ] Postpartum haemorrhage
- [ ] Bonding
- [ ] Communication with mother and family

Neonatology

- [ ] Routine examination of newborn
- [ ] Resuscitation of newborn/Apgar scoring
- [ ] Common abnormalities of the baby
- [ ] Jaundice
- [ ] Birth trauma
- [ ] Care and feeding of the newborn
- [ ] Respiratory distress syndrome
- [ ] Diabetes and its risks
- [ ] Low-birth-weight babies
- [ ] Preterm babies

Physiology of puerperium

- [ ] Breast-feeding
- [ ] Puerperal fever
- [ ] Puerperal depression
- [ ] Contraception advice
- [ ] Rubella vaccination
- [ ] Anti-D vaccination
- [ ] The 6-week check

Gynaecology

- [ ] History taking
- [ ] Examination of abdomen and pelvis
- [ ] Health education and promotion for women
- [ ] Physiology of menstrual cycle

☐ Congenital abnormalities
☐ Psychosexual counselling principles

Menstrual problems

☐ Amenorrhoea
☐ Menorrhagia
☐ Dysmenorrhoea
☐ Premenstrual syndrome
☐ Puberty
☐ The menopause/hormone replacement therapy

Pregnancy-related problems

☐ Abortions and habitual abortions
☐ Ectopic pregnancy
☐ Management of infertility (including IVF and GIFT)

Neoplasia

☐ Uterine
☐ Breast
☐ Ovarian
☐ Vaginal
☐ Vulval
☐ Cervical
☐ Cervical intraepithelial neoplasia and cervical smears
☐ Colposcopy techniques

Other gynaecological problems

☐ Sexually transmitted disease (including AIDS)
☐ Pelvic inflammatory disease
☐ Vaginal infections and discharge
☐ Vulval dystrophy
☐ Fibroids
☐ Endometriosis
☐ Prolapse
☐ Urinary tract problems in women
☐ Urinary incontinence
☐ Urodynamic studies
☐ Infections
☐ Common gynaecological operations

Family planning

- [ ] Failure rates, acceptability and motivation
- [ ] Natural methods
- [ ] Barrier methods: sheath/caps and diaphragms
- [ ] Spermicides
- [ ] Hormonal methods
- [ ] Combined pill
- [ ] Mini-pill
- [ ] Implants
- [ ] Injectables
- [ ] Post-coital contraception
- [ ] Intrauterine contraceptive device
- [ ] Sterilisation
- [ ] Terminations
- [ ] Recent advances
- [ ] 'Female condom'
- [ ] Luteinising hormone releasing hormone analogues
- [ ] Male pill
- [ ] GP protocol, including claim forms
- [ ] Family planning clinics

The Examination Day

Having passed a usually troubled and seemingly endless night, it is at last time to get up. Give yourself plenty of time.

It is important that you are comfortable during the exam, but remember that you will be seeing patients and it is important to be smart.

If you are taking the exam at a distant centre make sure you book your accommodation well in advance. It is not a good idea to travel a long distance on the day of the exam as hold-ups can and do occur which add unnecessary stress to the already anxious candidate. Remember that no allowance is made for late arrival.

After arriving at the place where you are staying make sure you know the way to the examination centre. If you have not been there before it can be very helpful to make the journey beforehand so that you then have an idea of the distance involved and the time it is likely to take. Be sure to allow extra time for rush-hour travel.

Pre-examination tension builds up however well prepared you are, so try to occupy your mind with non-related topics. If travelling by rail you will find that a novel passes the time admirably and prevents brooding. Never take textbooks, it is far too late for them to do any good; they may well cause confusion and add to your anxiety.

Check that you have all the documentation you need to be admitted to the exam. Leave in plenty of time to allow for unexpected delays. Aim to arrive at the centre 15–20 minutes before the exam starts, if you arrive too early the anxious chatter and cross-questioning between the other candidates can have an unnerving effect.

The examination is conducted in two parts, the Multiple Choice Question (MCQ) paper and the Objective Structured Clinical Examination (OSCE). In certain centres they may be run at different locations and coaches may be used to ferry the candidates between venues. Read the College instructions well in advance.

The MCQ paper and the OSCE paper are weighted equally, each offering the candidate a score of up to 50%. The pass mark for each part is a mean score −1 standard deviation. Candidates must pass both parts in order to pass the examination.

For the written examination you will be admitted to the examination room 10–15 minutes before the examination is due to start. Leave coats, brief-cases, etc. where indicated by the invigilators. Take your correct seat. There will be a card on the desk with a number on it which corresponds to the number on your admission card.

Read the instructions printed on the paper carefully. On the front cover you must print your full name in the boxes provided and add your signature in the marked space. Your candidate number should be written in the four squares provided.

Conclusion

Most candidates who fail, fail themselves. Errors of commission are much more common than errors of omission. It is hoped that the hints provided in this book will help you to avoid most pitfalls and will add a little extra 'finish' to your performance.

Good luck.

MCQ
Practice Exams

The Multiple Choice Question Paper

Multiple choice questions are the most consistent, reproducible and internally reliable method we have of testing recall of factual knowledge. Yet there is evidence that they are able to test more than simple factual recall; reasoning ability and understanding of basic facts, principles and concepts can also be assessed. A good MCQ paper will discriminate accurately between candidates on the basis of their knowledge of the topics being tested. It must be emphasised that the most important function of an MCQ paper of the type used in the DRCOG, is to rank candidates accurately and fairly according to their performance in that paper. Accurate ranking is the key phrase; this means that all MCQ examinations of this type are in a sense competitive.

The MCQ paper consists of 60 multiple choice questions in book form and will include a broad spectrum of questions in obstetrics, gynaecology, family planning, paediatrics and associated subjects.

Examination technique

The safest way to pass the DRCOG is to know the answers to all of the questions, but it is equally important to be able to transfer this knowledge accurately on to the answer sheet. All too often, candidates suffer through an inability to organise their time, through failure to read the instructions carefully, or through failure to read and understand the questions. First of all you must allocate your time with care. There are 60 questions to complete in two hours; this means two minutes per question. Make sure that you are getting through the exam at least at this pace or, if possible, a little quicker, thus allowing time at the end for revision and a re-think on some of the items that you have deferred.

It may be helpful for you to read through the whole paper first in order to get a feel for the total contents. Then you can go through the paper answering all the questions that you are sure of, ie immediate recall of information. Lastly go through the paper again slowly, answering all the questions that you can.

You must read the question (both stem and items) carefully. You should be quite clear that you know what you are being asked to do. Once you know

3

this, you should indicate your responses by marking the answer sheet boldly, correctly and clearly. Take great care not to mark the wrong boxes and think very carefully before making a mark on the computer answer sheet. Regard each item as being independent of every other item, each refers to a specific quantum of knowledge. The item (or the stem and the item taken together) make up a statement. You are required to indicate whether you regard this statement as 'True' or 'False'.

Marking your answer sheets

The answer sheet will be read by an automatic document reader, which transfers the information it reads to a computer. It must therefore be filled out in accordance with the instructions. A sample of the answer sheet, together with the instructions is available from the Royal College. Study the instructions carefully, well before the exam, the invigilators will also draw your attention to them at the time of the examination. You must first fill in your name on the answer sheet and then fill in your examination number. It is critical that this is filled in correctly with the 2B pencil provided.

As you go through the questions, you can either mark your answers immediately on the answer sheet, or you can mark them in the question book first of all, transferring them to the answer sheets at the end. However, if you adopt the second approach (as recommended by the Royal College) you must take great care not to run out of time, since you will not be allowed extra time to transfer marks to the answer sheet from the question book. The answer sheet must always be marked neatly and carefully according to the instructions given. Careless marking is probably one of the commonest causes of rejection of answer sheets by the document reader. You are, of course, at liberty to change your mind by erasing your original selection and selecting a new one. In this event, your erasure should be carefully, neatly and completely carried out.

Try to leave time to go over your answers again before the end, in particular going back over any difficult questions that you wish to think about in more detail. At the same time, you can check that you have marked the answer sheet correctly. However, repeated review of your answers may in the end be counter-productive, since answers that you were originally confident were absolutely correct, often look rather less convincing at a second, third, or fourth perusal. In this situation, first thoughts are usually best and too critical a revision might lead you into a state of confusion.

The marking system: to guess or not to guess

Each block correctly filled in scores +1, and each block incorrectly filled in scores 0. There is no longer a system of negative marking in this exam, thus it is in your best interest to answer every question. Try and guess if you do not know the answer, you will not be penalised if you get it wrong and you will gain a point if you get it right. No question should remain unanswered.

Trust the examiners

Do try to trust the examiners. Accept each question at its face value and do not look for hidden meanings, catches and ambiguities. Multiple choice questions are not designed to trick or confuse you, they are designed to test your knowledge of medicine. Do not look for problems that are not there, the obvious meaning of a statement is the correct one and the one that you should read.

To repeat the most important points of technique:

1.   Read the question carefully and be sure you understand it.

2.   Mark your responses clearly and accurately.

3.   Do not leave any questions unanswered, there is nothing to be lost by guessing.

4.   The best way to obtain a good mark is to have as wide a knowledge as possible of the topics being tested in the examination.

Royal College of Obstetricians and Gynaecologists
Diploma Examination (DRCOG)

CANDIDATE NUMBER

SURNAME
(FAMILY NAME)

OTHER
NAME(S)

Please use HB pencil. Rub out all errors thoroughly.
Mark lozenges like ▬ NOT like ✓ X O

T = True
F = False

IMPORTANT NOTES

1. When you have finished, check that you have NOT left any blanks.

2. Erasures should be left clean, with no smudges where possible. (The document reading machine will accept the darkest response for each item).

CHECK THAT YOU HAVE ANSWERED EVERY ITEM TRUE OR FALSE

Sample computer marking sheet reproduced with the kind permission of the Royal College of Obstetricians and Gynaecologists.

MCQ Practice Exam Instructions

It is recommended that you should work on these three practice examinations as though they were real examinations. In other words, time yourself to spend no more than two hours on each practice exam and do not obtain help from books, notes, or persons while working on each test. Plan to take a practice exam at a time when you will be undisturbed for a minimum of two hours. Choose a well-lit location, free from distractions, keep your desk clear of other books or papers, and have a clock or watch clearly visible.

As you work through each question in this book be sure to mark a tick or cross (True or False) against each answer option. If you do not know the answer then leave the answer box blank. (In the exam as there is no negative marking you must answer *all* the questions.)

When you have completed the paper you can mark your own answers with the help of the answers and explanations given at the end of the exam. Do not be tempted to look at the questions before sitting down to take the test as it will not then represent a mock exam.

MCQ Practice Exam 1

60 Questions: time allowed 2 hours. Indicate your answers clearly by putting a tick or cross against each answer option.

1. **The following statements about fetal cardiotocography are true:**

   ☐ **A** Fetal heart rate decreases with increasing gestational age
   ☐ **B** The normal baseline heart rate in late pregnancy is between 120 and 150 bpm
   ☐ **C** Baseline tachycardia can be associated with maternal fever
   ☐ **D** Heart rate variability increases with increasing gestational age
   ☐ **E** Late decelerations and reduced variability are associated with fetal hypoxia

2. **Dyspareunia**

   ☐ **A** is classed as superficial when pain occurs after penetration
   ☐ **B** can be caused by a urethral caruncle
   ☐ **C** is associated with vaginal lactobacilli
   ☐ **D** is associated with atrophic vaginitis
   ☐ **E** may require a laparoscopy to help in the diagnosis

3. **Anti-D prophylaxis should be given to all nonsensitised rhesus-D-negative women after the following events in the 3rd trimester:**

   ☐ **A** Eclamptic fit
   ☐ **B** HELLP (haemolysis, elevated liver enzymes and a low platelet count) syndrome
   ☐ **C** Transvaginal scan
   ☐ **D** Premature labour
   ☐ **E** Abdominal trauma

4. **Endometrial biopsy**

   ☐ **A** should be restricted to women over the age of 35 years
   ☐ **B** should be carried out before the commencement of hormone replacement therapy
   ☐ **C** always requires an anaesthetic
   ☐ **D** is mandatory in women on unopposed oestrogen who have an intact uterus
   ☐ **E** is mainly used to detect endometrial polyps

5. **The following are diagnostic tests for Down's syndrome:**

   ☐ **A** Chorionic villus sampling
   ☐ **B** α-fetoprotein testing
   ☐ **C** A combination of α-fetoprotein, β-human chorionic gonadotrophin and oestriol testing in maternal serum
   ☐ **D** Amniocentesis
   ☐ **E** Ultrasound scanning at 12 weeks' gestation

6. **The following statements about pelvic inflammatory disease (PID) are true:**

   ☐ **A** It is considered a sexually transmitted disease
   ☐ **B** It has an incidence of about 1 per 1000 in all women between the ages of 15 and 39
   ☐ **C** About 15% of all females will have had PID by the age of 30
   ☐ **D** It is now widely accepted as polymicrobial in origin
   ☐ **E** Chronic PID is a rare complaint

7. **Breech presentation may be due to**

   ☐ **A** bicornuate uterus
   ☐ **B** hydrocephalus
   ☐ **C** polyhydramnios
   ☐ **D** placenta praevia
   ☐ **E** prematurity

8. **The progestogen-only pill method of contraception is particularly indicated in:**

   ☐ **A** Women over 35 who smoke
   ☐ **B** Women with endometriosis
   ☐ **C** During lactation
   ☐ **D** Patients with hyperemesis
   ☐ **E** Patients with diabetes

9. **The following recommendations about the management of a woman with suspected varicella contact in pregnancy are true:**

☐ **A** If a pregnant woman has had a significant contact and no previous history of varicella then check the varicella immunoglobulin G (IgG) in the serum

☐ **B** If the pregnant woman is not immune to varicella zoster and the infection occurs before 20 weeks' gestation then she should be given varicella zoster IgG as soon as possible

☐ **C** Detection of IgG in maternal serum indicates primary varicella zoster infection

☐ **D** If the woman develops primary varicella in the first 20 weeks of pregnancy then she has a 2% risk of a congenital varicella infection

☐ **E** If there is no previous history of varicella and the contact occurs after 20 weeks there is no risk of congenital varicella infection

10. **Amenorrhoea can be caused by**

☐ **A** hypogonadotrophic hypogonadism
☐ **B** anaemia
☐ **C** hypoprolactinaemia
☐ **D** Turner's syndrome
☐ **E** Asherman's syndrome

11. **Patients from Africa have an increased incidence of**

☐ **A** fibroids
☐ **B** endometriosis
☐ **C** ectopic pregnancy
☐ **D** severe pre-eclampsia
☐ **E** postmenopausal osteoporosis

12. **Ovulation can be induced by the use of the following:**

☐ **A** Clomiphene citrate
☐ **B** Ethinyloestradiol
☐ **C** Medroxyprogesterone acetate
☐ **D** Human chorionic gonadotrophin
☐ **E** Human menopausal gonadotrophin

13. Anti-D should be given

- ☐ **A** to all cases of threatened abortion
- ☐ **B** to a rhesus-negative woman who has just delivered
- ☐ **C** to a rhesus-negative woman two weeks postpartum
- ☐ **D** during an *in vitro* fertilisation cycle
- ☐ **E** at the time of amniocentesis in rhesus-negative women

14. The use of progestogen-only contraceptives is governed by the following considerations:

- ☐ **A** Ovulation is not always inhibited
- ☐ **B** Protection against pregnancy is as good as with the combined pill
- ☐ **C** There is a substantial risk in older women of thromboembolic phenomena
- ☐ **D** Uterine bleeding may become irregular
- ☐ **E** The dose of progestogen is much larger than in the combined pill

15. Magnesium sulphate

- ☐ **A** is used in the management of intrauterine growth retardation
- ☐ **B** is used in the prevention of eclampsia
- ☐ **C** can cause loss of deep tendon reflexes
- ☐ **D** can cause loss of respiratory depression
- ☐ **E** has a therapeutic range between 30 and 40 mmol/l

16. A pulmonary embolism should be suspected if there is

- ☐ **A** a painful calf
- ☐ **B** haemoptysis
- ☐ **C** pyrexia
- ☐ **D** hypertension
- ☐ **E** a dry cough

17. **The following statements of advice on preventing deep vein thrombosis for pregnant women travelling by air are true:**

   ☐ **A** There is good, direct, evidence-based data to guide thrombo-prophylactic advice for pregnant air travellers
   ☐ **B** An increase in body mass index is not an additional risk factor
   ☐ **C** Women with a past history or strong family history of deep vein thrombosis should minimise alcohol and coffee consumption
   ☐ **D** Women with multiple pregnancy on a long-haul flight should consider low-molecular-weight heparin on the day of travel and the day after
   ☐ **E** Low-dose aspirin 75 mg per day for three days before travel and on the day of travel is an acceptable alternative in those unable to take low-molecular-weight heparin

18. **The following statements as to the cause of subfertility are true:**

   ☐ **A** Endometriosis is found in about 25% of cases
   ☐ **B** Ovulatory failure accounts for about 20% of cases
   ☐ **C** Sperm defects are found in about 5% of couples
   ☐ **D** Tubal damage is the most common cause in females
   ☐ **E** A cause is found after standard investigation in about 70% of cases

19. **Recognised causes of neonatal fits include**

   ☐ **A** hypoglycaemia
   ☐ **B** birth trauma
   ☐ **C** meningitis
   ☐ **D** Down's syndrome
   ☐ **E** bottle feeding

20. **The following statements about semen analysis are true:**

   ☐ **A** Normal volume is between 2 and 5 ml
   ☐ **B** Aspermia may be due to retrograde ejaculation
   ☐ **C** Asthenospermia means decreased motility
   ☐ **D** Motility is usually greater than 40%
   ☐ **E** Analysis should be performed 10–12 days after the last ejaculation

21. Causes of anovulation include

- ☐ **A** hypoprolactinaemia
- ☐ **B** polycystic ovarian syndrome
- ☐ **C** premature menopause
- ☐ **D** hypothalamic hypogonadism
- ☐ **E** wedge resection of the ovaries

22. Endometriosis

- ☐ **A** is defined as functional endometrial tissue outside the uterine cavity
- ☐ **B** histological examination of deposits is essential to confirm the presence of glands and stroma
- ☐ **C** is always symptomatic
- ☐ **D** has an incidence of about 10% which is increasing
- ☐ **E** is always associated with subfertility

23. Primary cytomegalovirus infection in pregnancy may cause the following in the fetus

- ☐ **A** Microcephaly
- ☐ **B** Blood dyscrasias
- ☐ **C** Myocarditis
- ☐ **D** Pneumonia
- ☐ **E** Enterocolitis

24. Reversal of sterilisation

- ☐ **A** is requested by about 10% of patients
- ☐ **B** has an ectopic rate of about 3%
- ☐ **C** if a Filshie clip has been applied, is successful in approximately 70% of cases
- ☐ **D** has an increased rate of success when an operating microscope is used
- ☐ **E** should only be considered if the patient's serum follicle-stimulating hormone level is >20 IU/l

25. The following are relative contraindications for laparoscopy being performed:

- ☐ **A** A positive pregnancy test
- ☐ **B** Previous pulmonary embolism
- ☐ **C** Chronic tuberculous peritonitis
- ☐ **D** A diaphragmatic hernia
- ☐ **E** Previous hysterectomy

26. In the healthy neonate

☐ **A** the onset of physiological jaundice is between the sixth and eighth day
☐ **B** the bowel is sterile at birth
☐ **C** urine is not normally passed until 24 hours after birth
☐ **D** the respiratory rate is in the region of 25–35 per minute
☐ **E** the ductus arteriosus closes functionally within an hour of birth

27. Endometrial carcinoma

☐ **A** is more common in obese patients
☐ **B** is a squamous carcinoma in the majority of cases
☐ **C** is more common in diabetic patients
☐ **D** can be excluded if a cervical smear is normal
☐ **E** is more common in postmenopausal women receiving cyclical oestrogen and progestogen hormone replacement therapy

28. Cephalopelvic disproportion

☐ **A** exists when the capacity of the birth canal is insufficient for safe vaginal delivery of the fetus with a cephalic presentation
☐ **B** can usually be diagnosed antenatally by abdominal palpation
☐ **C** may be associated with non-engagement of the head at term
☐ **D** is accurately diagnosed by X-ray pelvimetry
☐ **E** often occurs with a brow presentation

29. Polyhydramnios may be due to

☐ **A** Potter's syndrome
☐ **B** oesophageal atresia
☐ **C** an open neural tube defect
☐ **D** Turner's syndrome
☐ **E** ovarian hyperstimulation syndrome

30. Preterm birth

☐ **A** is defined as delivery of an infant between 24 and 37 completed weeks
☐ **B** occurs in about 1% of all births
☐ **C** is due to multiple pregnancy in 6% of cases
☐ **D** is associated with congenital uterine abnormalities
☐ **E** can be prevented in 70% of occasions by tocolytics

31. Bacterial vaginosis is associated with the following complications of pregnancy:

☐ **A** Gestational diabetes
☐ **B** Pre-eclampsia
☐ **C** Prolonged pregnancy
☐ **D** Low birth weight
☐ **E** Preterm labour

32. At antenatal booking

☐ **A** women should have been informed of the hospital's antenatal plan and advised to follow it
☐ **B** should be advised not to wear a seat belt
☐ **C** should have their body mass index measured
☐ **D** should have a psychiatric history taken
☐ **E** should be encouraged to have HIV screening

33. The following advice should be given to pregnant women:

☐ **A** Sexual activity should be reduced
☐ **B** Maternal smoking should be reduced because it reduces average birth weight
☐ **C** Excessive alcohol consumption by the mother can be associated with fetal growth retardation
☐ **D** Women with previous growth-retarded infants should not continue to work during any future pregnancies
☐ **E** Folic acid should be taken in a dose of 4 mg/day by all pregnant women

34. The following statements about pelvic inflammatory disease (PID) are true:

☐ **A** Is often due to *Mycoplasma hominis*
☐ **B** About 20% of women who have it are infertile
☐ **C** About 20% of women who have it develop chronic pelvic pain
☐ **D** Has an increased instance in women with higher socioeconomic circumstances.
☐ **E** Has an increased incidence in African/Afro-Caribbean women

35. Giving iron supplements in pregnancy to prevent anaemia

- ☐ **A** reduces the incidence of proteinuric hypertension
- ☐ **B** reduces the incidence of antepartum haemorrhage
- ☐ **C** reduces the incidence of maternal infection
- ☐ **D** decreases the incidence of preterm delivery
- ☐ **E** decreases the incidence of intrauterine growth retardation

36. Regarding ovarian hyperstimulation syndrome:

- ☐ **A** Ovarian hyperstimulation syndrome (OHSS) is an iatrogenic condition
- ☐ **B** If no pregnancy occurs, the syndrome will typically resolve within two months
- ☐ **C** The treatment of OHSS is often careful observation
- ☐ **D** Severe OHSS is characterised by the presence of free intraperitoneal fluid, pleural effusions and oliguria
- ☐ **E** The incidence of mild and moderate forms of OHSS is <1% of all females undergoing ovulation induction

37. Regarding postnatal mental illnesses:

- ☐ **A** The postnatal blues occurs in 50–80% of all women who give birth
- ☐ **B** Postnatal psychosis affects 10–20% of women in the post-partum period
- ☐ **C** The postnatal depression occurs in 0.2% of all women who give birth
- ☐ **D** 20% is the postnatal psychosis recurrence rate in the next pregnancy
- ☐ **E** The blues are characterised by a significant mood swinging and a disturbance in perception

38. Electronic fetal monitoring:

- ☐ **A** Normal fetal heart baseline rate is between 120 and 150 beats per minute
- ☐ **B** The cardiotocography recording speeds vary from 2–5 cm per minute
- ☐ **C** Ritodrine is associated with a reduced fetal heart rate
- ☐ **D** Magnesium sulphate causes a decrease in fetal heart rate variability
- ☐ **E** The prevalence of cerebral palsy from intrapartum events is about 1%

39. The following statements are true:

- [ ] **A** By 2025 the number of people aged over 65 will have risen from 420 million in 2000 to 825 million
- [ ] **B** The definition of the menopause is 'the permanent cessation of menstruation resulting from the loss of pituitary activity'
- [ ] **C** The climacteric is the phase which marks the transition from the reproductive to the non-reproductive state
- [ ] **D** Premature menopause is stated to have occurred if menses ceases before the age of 47
- [ ] **E** The menopause is caused by ovarian failure

40. A 38-year-old woman presents with menorrhagia and dysmenorrhoea four years after being sterilised by the Filshie clip method. She complains that she requires three boxes of tampons for each period. No abnormality was found on pelvic examination.

- [ ] **A** The amount of sanitary protection correlates well with menstrual blood loss
- [ ] **B** The woman's subjective assessment of her blood loss is likely to be reasonably accurate
- [ ] **C** Her menstrual problems are caused by the sterilisation procedure
- [ ] **D** The only effective treatment is a hysterectomy and bilateral salpingo-oophorectomy
- [ ] **E** Anovulation is a likely cause

41. The following factors positively influence high birth weight

- [ ] **A** Maternal growth hormone
- [ ] **B** Prolonged pregnancy (>294 days)
- [ ] **C** Fetal hyperinsulinaemia
- [ ] **D** Primiparity
- [ ] **E** Social class

42. Possible causes of an unstable lie include

- [ ] **A** polyhydramnios
- [ ] **B** prematurity
- [ ] **C** uterine abnormality
- [ ] **D** placenta praevia
- [ ] **E** fibroid uterus

43. A hysterosalpingogram

- [ ] **A** confirms tubal function
- [ ] **B** can be used to diagnose uterine adhesions
- [ ] **C** is a diagnostic test for ectopic pregnancy
- [ ] **D** when performed, should be accompanied by a prophylactic antibiotic
- [ ] **E** is useful in the diagnosis of the effect of fibroids in infertility

44. Bilateral salpingo-oophorectomy at the time of hysterectomy

- [ ] **A** eliminates premenstrual syndrome
- [ ] **B** is technically more difficult than a hysterectomy
- [ ] **C** should never be performed in women under the age of 35
- [ ] **D** is the treatment of choice in stage 1 endometrial carcinoma
- [ ] **E** always requires the use of post-operative hormone replacement therapy

45. The following statement about vulvovaginal candidiasis are true:

- [ ] **A** Thrush affects about 25% of women at least once in their life time
- [ ] **B** *Candida albicans* is a commensal in the human genital and digestive tracts
- [ ] **C** *Candida glabrata* causes 75–80% of vulvovaginal candidiasis
- [ ] **D** Bubble bath causes vaginal thrush
- [ ] **E** A raised pH of the vagina is diagnostic

46. Dysmenorrhoea

- [ ] **A** is called primary if it occurs with ovulation
- [ ] **B** if it is primary, is associated with an abnormal level of prostaglandins
- [ ] **C** is called secondary when an organic cause is found
- [ ] **D** if secondary, may be caused by pelvic inflammatory disease
- [ ] **E** if primary, the oral contraceptive pill is useful treatment

47. The following statements about twin pregnancy are true:

- [ ] **A** Monozygotic twins occur at a fairly constant rate
- [ ] **B** It is associated with an increased risk of placenta praevia
- [ ] **C** Reducing the number of embryos replaced during IVF reduces the twinning risk
- [ ] **D** The risk of dizygotic twins decreases with increasing maternal age and parity
- [ ] **E** It is associated with an increased risk of gestational diabetes

48. Tubal patency is required for the following methods of assisted conception:

- [ ] **A** Intrauterine insemination
- [ ] **B** *In vitro* fertilisation
- [ ] **C** Donor insemination
- [ ] **D** Gamete intrafallopian transfer
- [ ] **E** Ovum donation

49. Intrauterine contraceptive devices

- [ ] **A** lead to an increase in the number of leukocytes in the endometrium and tubal fluid
- [ ] **B** cause a decrease in local prostaglandins
- [ ] **C** containing copper are toxic to sperm and the blastocyst
- [ ] **D** can contain a slow-release progestogen
- [ ] **E** are usually inert

50. The volume of amniotic fluid

- [ ] **A** is independent of fetal urine production
- [ ] **B** may be accurately measured by ultrasound
- [ ] **C** is excessive in severe rhesus disease
- [ ] **D** increases following amniocentesis
- [ ] **E** is reduced in severe pre-eclampsia

51. The following statements about starting combined oral contraceptives (COC) are true:

- [ ] **A** Starting on day one of menstruation extra precautions are required for seven days
- [ ] **B** If postpartum and not lactating the combined oral contraceptive pill can be started on day 21
- [ ] **C** During lactation the combined oral contraceptive pill can be started after 49 days
- [ ] **D** After an induced early abortion or miscarriage a combined oral contraceptive pill can be started the next day
- [ ] **E** The combined oral contraceptive pill can be started post-progestogen-only pill on the first day of a period and no extra precautions are required

52. The following are recognised causes of jaundice in the newborn:

- ☐ **A** A cephalohaematoma following a ventouse delivery
- ☐ **B** Physiological causes that occur around day seven
- ☐ **C** Infection
- ☐ **D** Rhesus incompatibility
- ☐ **E** Hypothyroidism with jaundice occurring in the first two days

53. In breech presentation

- ☐ **A** the perinatal morbidity is greater in the extended than in the flexed type
- ☐ **B** meconium is a reliable indicator of fetal distress
- ☐ **C** variable decelerations of fetal heart rate are a likely finding during intrapartum monitoring
- ☐ **D** breech extraction is the method of choice for a safe vaginal delivery
- ☐ **E** the obstetric forceps are not necessary in multiparous patients

54. The side-effects of the following drugs are correct:

- ☐ **A** Oestrogens – weight gain
- ☐ **B** Acyclovir – rises in bilirubin and liver enzymes
- ☐ **C** Fluconazole – nausea and abdominal discomfort
- ☐ **D** Bromocriptine – hypertension
- ☐ **E** Danazol – dry skin

55. Risk factors for pre-eclampsia include

- ☐ **A** obesity
- ☐ **B** previous severe pre-eclampsia
- ☐ **C** underweight and short
- ☐ **D** age between 25 and 35 years
- ☐ **E** chronic renal disease

56. The following statements about hydatidiform mole are correct:

- ☐ **A** There is a decreased incidence with increasing age
- ☐ **B** It may present with pre-eclampsia
- ☐ **C** It gives a typical ultrasound appearance
- ☐ **D** It is monitored post-evacuation by urinary oestriol levels
- ☐ **E** It is treated by methotrexate

57. Ovarian cancer:

- [ ] **A** Most women with early-stage cancer of the ovary do not have any symptoms
- [ ] **B** Ovarian cancer may present as a postmenopausal bleeding
- [ ] **C** The incidence increases with age to a peak in the 40–50 years old group
- [ ] **D** Normal CA125 levels exclude ovarian cancer
- [ ] **E** CA125 may increase in pelvic inflammatory disease

58. *Why Mothers Die 1997–1999* 'Report on confidential enquiry into maternal deaths in the United Kingdom' shows that maternal mortality rates increase among:

- [ ] **A** Women from the traditional travelling community
- [ ] **B** Women from ethnic groups other than white
- [ ] **C** Young women under 18 years of age
- [ ] **D** Women with increased maternal age
- [ ] **E** Women with high parity

59. If a pregnant woman comes into contact with rubella

- [ ] **A** the majority of women will have an abnormal fetus
- [ ] **B** a blood test taken immediately showing IgG antibodies means the fetus will not be affected
- [ ] **C** the baby may have high-tone deafness
- [ ] **D** gammaglobulin should be given as soon as possible
- [ ] **E** the highest risk of fetal damage occurs at four weeks' gestation

60. Predisposing factors for uterovaginal prolapse:

- [ ] **A** High parity
- [ ] **B** The menopause
- [ ] **C** Ascites
- [ ] **D** Previous treatment with large loop excision of transformation zone (LLETZ)
- [ ] **E** Chronic cough

MCQ Practice Exam 1: Answers and Teaching Notes

1. **A C**

   Understanding cardiotocograms is important. Baseline tachycardias can be associated with drugs, prematurity, hypoxia, or maternal pyrexia. Baseline bradycardia (90–120 bpm) is significant if there are also decelerations or decreased variability. It can very rarely be due to congenital heart problems. Severe bradycardia (<90 bpm) is usually associated with a severely compromised fetus. Chronic hypoxia causes a loss of baseline variability. Early deceleration begins with the onset of a contraction and quickly returns to the baseline before the end of the contraction. It is usually associated with compression of the fetal head and is not an indication of fetal distress. On the other hand, late deceleration is associated with fetal hypoxia and is present when the low point of the deceleration occurs after the peak of the contraction with a slow rate of recovery of the fetal heart. Variable decelerations are sometimes difficult to interpret and can be associated with cord compression.

2. **B D E**

   Dyspareunia is pain or difficulty with intercourse. Superficial dyspareunia is defined as pain at the onset of penetration while deep dyspareunia is pain that occurs after penetration. Superficial dyspareunia can be associated with vulval, vaginal and urethral disease. Vaginal lactobacillus is a normal vaginal flora. Postmenopausal atrophic vaginitis responds well to local oestrogen therapy. Deep dyspareunia is often associated with pelvic pathology, such as pelvic inflammatory disease, endometriosis, ovarian cysts, uterine fibroids and ectopic pregnancy.

3. **E**

   The following are potentially sensitising events during pregnancy:

   - Invasive prenatal diagnosis, eg chorionic villus sampling, amniocentesis, fetal blood sampling
   - Antepartum haemorrhage
   - External cephalic version of fetus
   - Abdominal trauma
   - Intrauterine death

4. A D

The main purpose of endometrial biopsy is the early detection of endometrial hyperplasia or malignancy. It does not reduce menstrual flow. Biopsies should be restricted to those women over the age of 35 as the prevalence of endometrial carcinoma is so uncommon in younger women. Before starting hormone replacement therapy there is no need to assess the endometrium routinely unless, of course, there is unexplained abnormal vaginal bleeding. Nowadays with different out-patient procedures including pipelles and varbra samplings there is usually no need to perform a general anaesthetic. Women with a uterus should not receive unopposed oestrogens because there is an increased risk of endometrial carcinoma and are in need of investigation. Flexible out-patient hysteroscopy with or without endometrial sampling and/or scanning is now an acceptable method of assessing the endometrial cavity.

5. A D

Note the term 'diagnostic'. Biochemistry and USS are useful as screening tests.

6. A D

PID is considered to be a sexually transmitted infection because sexual intercourse provides the necessary damage and as the endometrium is always affected it is concluded that the infection ascends. The incidence is around 10 per 1000 in all women between the ages of 15 and 39, but may increase to 20 per 1000 in the 15–24 age group. PID is widely accepted as polymicrobial in origin. *Chlamydia trachomatis* and *Neisseria gonorrhoea* are the organisms usually transmitted, but others, such as *Mycoplasma hominis*, *Mycoplasma genitalis* and *Ureaplasma urealyticum*, can be involved. The endogenous flora of the lower genital tract often act as secondary pathogens. These include group B streptococci, *Escherichia coli*, *Gardnerella vaginalis*, *Clostridium* spp., *Actinomyces* and *Bacteroides* spp. Chronic PID is an extremely frequent complaint with sufferers from a first episode running six to ten times the risk of suffering from further episodes. There is a 1:6 chance of tubal infertility, a seven-fold increase of ectopic pregnancy, a 1:5 chance of deep dyspareunia and a 4:5 chance of menstrual disturbances.

7. **All true**

There are many causes of breech presentation:

1. Maternal causes:
- grand multiparity
- uterine abnormalities, including bicornuate uterus
- pelvic tumours, including ovarian cysts and fibroids
- severe bony pelvic abnormality

2. Fetal problems:
- prematurity, the prevalence of breech presentation decreases from about 15% at 29–32 weeks' gestation to 3–4% at delivery
- multiple pregnancy
- fetal abnormality which could be associated with polyhydramnios, oligohydramnios or hydrocephalus

3. Placenta praevia.

8. **A C D E**

With the present evidence progestogen-only pill can be continued in smokers. Progestogen-only pill should not be chosen in preference to the combined oral contraceptive pill in patients with endometriosis as it does not reliably suppress endogenous oestrogen. Diabetics tolerate the progestogen-only pill resulting in good compliance. In obese women efficacy is a concern. As a working rule Professor John Guillebaud in his book *Contraception – Your Questions Answered* states – 'Contraindications to or side-effects with the combined oral contraceptive pill, and a hormonal method is preferred? Try the progestogen-only pill'.

9. **A B D E**

At least 85% of women have had varicella and will have a positive IgG. Detection of IgM in maternal serum indicates primary varicella infection. Referral to a specialist centre for detailed ultrasound examination at 16–20 weeks' gestation or five weeks after infection which ever is sooner should be considered.

Neonatal ophthalmic examination should be organised at birth. If the infection occurs after 20 weeks there is still a risk of maternal varicella pneumonia.

If the pregnant woman is in the second half of pregnancy and is seen less than 24 hours after the development of a varicella rash then administration of acyclovir may be expected to reduce the severity and duration of the illness. There are theoretical concerns about teratogenesis when acyclovir is used in the first trimester but these have not been confirmed. Delay of delivery by 5–7 days after the onset of maternal illness allows for the passive transfer of antibodies. Detection of IgM in maternal serum indicates varicella infection.

10. A D E

Primary amenorrhoea can be due to several causes:

- Constitutional/idiopathic. This accounts for about 15% of the cases. In these instances the gonadotrophins are usually low.
- Gonadal failure. These include pure gonadal dysgenesis, Turner's syndrome and non-dysgenetic failure. Elevated serum gonadotrophins are present and this occurs in about 45% of cases.
- Hypothalamic pituitary dysfunction, such as hypogonadotrophic hypogonadism (Kallmann's syndrome). In these instances the serum gonadotrophins are low; they account for about 25% of the cause of delayed puberty.
- Defective steroid synthesis. This can account for primary amenorrhoea and delayed puberty as well as chronic illnesses and malnutrition. In both these instances low gonadotrophins are present.

Causes of secondary amenorrhoea are as follows:

- Physiological causes, pregnancies, menopause.
- Gonadotrophin abnormalities, hyperprolactinaemia, structural problems in the pituitary, hypogonadotrophic hypogonadism, polycystic ovarian syndrome, weight loss, chronic illness and psychogenic causes.
- Primary ovarian failure, premature menopause, resistant ovarian syndrome, genital tract abnormalities, such as Asherman's syndrome, and other endocrinopathies, eg thyroid dysfunction (hypothyroidism).

11. A C D

African patients have a different incidence of disease. Fibroids are increased, although endometriosis is said to be relatively rare. Ectopic pregnancy does appear to be increased, but this is probably associated with tubal disease following pelvic inflammatory disease. Postmenopausal osteoporosis is less common.

12. A D E

Clomiphene citrate has oestrogenic and anti-oestrogenic properties. It should not be given to patients who are ovulating because it will interfere with the oestradiol receptors in the endometrium, raise basal luteinising hormone and possibly affect the production of cervical mucus. Sometimes, to induce ovulation, human chorionic gonadotrophin can be given along with clomiphene. Human menopausal gonadotrophin is a mixture of follicle-stimulating hormone and luteinising hormone which has an action mainly on the follicular growth. Ovum release and luteinisation can then be achieved by use of human chorionic gonadotrophin.

13. B E

All cases of threatened abortion do not need anti-D as the woman may not be rhesus negative. There is no indication to give anti-D during an in vitro fertilisation cycle. Even in Rhesus negative women Anti-D is no longer necessary in women with threatened miscarriage unless there is a large amount of vaginal bleeding.

14. A D

The progestogen-only pill is less effective than the combined pill but there are no serious adverse effects. The dose of progestogen is much smaller than that in the combined pill. The newer desogestrel pill does cause anovulation and is claimed to be as effective as the combined oral contraceptive pill.

15. B C D

Following the Collaborative Eclampsia Trial women treated with magnesium sulphate have fewer recurrent seizures compared with women treated with diazepam or phenytoin. It appears to reduce cerebral vasospasm. Monitoring of therapy should include hourly measurement of the patellar reflex and respiratory rate or oxygen saturation. If reflexes become absent then magnesium should be discontinued until their return. Respiratory depression should be treated with calcium gluconate.

16. B C D E

A painful, tender calf should lead to suspicions of a deep vein thrombosis which may be associated with a pulmonary embolism. The signs and symptoms of pulmonary embolism can easily be missed. Typically, there is a pleuritic pain associated with haemoptysis, dyspnoea and, in severe cases, it may be associated with hypertension. Other suspicious features include a dry cough, pyrexia and tachycardia.

17. C D E

Summary table of the RCOG, Scientific Advisory Committee Advice on preventing thromboembolism in pregnant women travelling by air.

Any gestation and up to 6 weeks postpartum	Short-haul flight (up to 4 hours)	Long-haul flight (4 hours or more)
No additional risk factors	Calf exercise; move around cabin; avoid dehydration; minimise alcohol and coffee consumption.	Calf exercise; move around cabin; avoid dehydration; minimise alcohol and coffee consumption; well-fitting elastic compression stockings.
Additional risk factors[a]	Calf exercise; move around cabin; avoid dehydration; minimise alcohol and coffee consumption; well-fitting elastic below-knee compression stockings.	Calf exercise; move around cabin; avoid dehydration; minimise alcohol and coffee consumption; well-fitting elastic below-knee compression stockings; low-molecular-weight heparin[b] on day of travel (pre-flight) and day after.

Weight $\geq$ 100 kg or BMI at booking $\geq$ 30+

Multiple pregnancy

Thrombophilia

Past personal or strong family history

Medical disorders with increased risk of deep vein thrombosis

[a] Women with additional risk factors may need to seek appropriate medical advice; some, for instance will already be on thromboprophylatic medication.

[b] Thromboprophylactic doses are 5000 units dalteparin or 40 mg enoxaparin. (Low-dose aspirin (75 mg per day for 3 days before travel and on day of travel) is an acceptable alternative in those unable to take low-molecular-weight heparin.)

18. **B E**

The main causes of infertility are shown below. Remember that some couples may have more than one cause.

Unexplained	30%
Sperm defects	25%
Ovulatory failure	20%
Tubal damage	15%
Others	10%
Endometriosis	5%
Mucus defects	5%
Other male problems	2%
Coital failure	2%

19. **A B C**

Fits may be associated with many different problems. These include:

- hypoglycaemia
- birth trauma
- asphyxia
- congenital structural abnormalities of the brain
- meningitis.

20. **A B C D**

A semen sample should be collected after a minimum of three days' and a maximum of five days' abstinence. The sample should be brought to the laboratory within one hour of production and examined as soon as possible. Normal semen parameters are:

- Volume >2–6 ml
- Density >20 × 10^6/ml
- Motility >40% forward progression after two hours
- Morphology >20% normal
- White blood cells <1 × 10^6 ml

21. **B C D**

Hyperprolactinaemia is associated with anovulation. Raised serum prolactin interferes with the hypothalamic release of gonadotrophin-releasing hormone. Hyperprolactinaemia may be due to an adenoma of the pituitary or may possibly be related to drugs, especially the phenothiazines. Women with polycystic ovarian syndrome may present with infrequent periods or no periods at all. They are often, but not always, obese with hirsutism and acne. Strenuous exercise or excessive weight loss may suggest a hypothalamic cause with a history of amenorrhoea. The wedge resection used to be a treatment for poly-cycstic ovarian syndrome. Electrodiathermy is now becoming an acceptable treatment of polycystic ovarian infertility.

22. A D

Endometriosis is the presence of functional endometrial tissue outside the uterine cavity and can also occur outside the pelvic cavity (it has been known to occur in the umbilicus or even abdominal scars). Ideally, histology should confirm the diagnosis. Adenomyosis occurs when endometrial tissue lies within the myometrium and is thus a histological diagnosis that can only be made at hysterectomy. There does appear to be an increasing instance of endometriosis in general. Incidence increases with age, with a peak around the ages of 40–45. It is estimated that 10% of menstruating Caucasians have endometriosis. They may be totally asymptomatic or may have marked symptoms. It is interesting that the extent of the disease is not correlated to the symptoms. Endometriosis is associated with infertility but may not **always** be. Endometriosis can cause anatomical distortion and this is usually with severe cases. Mild endometriosis with peritoneal deposits may upset fertilisation and there is now evidence that ablating these areas may be beneficial – drug therapy does not improve conception rates.

23. A B D

Primary cytomegalovirus (CMV) infection during pregnancy may affect both the placenta and the fetus in up to 50% of cases. The prognosis of the infection in the fetus is not accurately known, but it is thought that such infection may produce microcephaly, choroido-retinitis, eighth nerve damage, pneumonia, hepatosplenomegaly, anaemia (sometimes haemolytic with jaundice) and intrauterine growth retardation. Myocarditis and enterocolitis are not usually associated with CMV infection.

24. B C D

The following patients are most likely to request reversal of sterilisation:

- A patient who was sterilised before the age of 30
- A patient who is in an unstable relationship
- A patient from a lower socioeconomic class
- A patient who was sterilised immediately after a pregnancy or during a termination of pregnancy
- A patient who has neurotic traits

Up to 60% of women requesting sterilisation reversal want children by another partner. The success rate does depend on the method of sterilisation and clip sterilisation reversal is easier than that following diathermy to the tubes. The ectopic rate after any reversal of sterilisation is about 3%. Most surgeons find that magnification helps and use of an operating microscope is ideal. A raised follicle-stimulating hormone indicates ovarian malfunction and reduced fertility, it needs to be repeated and then counselling should be offered – reversal may not be appropriate. Do not forget to also discuss *in vitro* fertilisation as an alternative.

25. C D
Laparoscopy is now being used more and more and, therefore, the contraindications are decreasing. Chronic tuberculous peritonitis is a contraindication because this is associated with quite marked abdominal adhesions and, therefore, perforation of the bowel is unrecognised. However, other previous abdominal surgery is not a contraindication. A laparoscopy is a regular method of detecting an ectopic pregnancy and is not, therefore, contraindicated in a pregnancy. In the advanced stages of pregnancy it is obviously contraindicated due to the damage that may be caused.

26. B D E
Physiological jaundice in a healthy baby appears after the first 48 hours of life, reaches a peak by about the fourth day and disappears within 7–10 days. The bowel is usually sterile at birth but is rapidly colonised by organisms, including those encountered along the birth canal and perineum. Urine is seen to be passed *in utero* on ultrasound and is frequently passed at or soon after birth. The respiratory rate is usually less than 60 per minute at rest, 25–35 being usual. Constriction of the ductus arteriosus is brought about by the direct effect on the vessel wall of raising the arteriolar $p(O_2)$ with ventilation of the lungs at birth. There is probably a rapid partial closure soon after birth followed by a more gradual closure during the course of several days.

27. A C
Obesity is associated with an increased level of unopposed oestrogens. Endometrial carcinoma is usually an adenocarcinoma and a negative cervical smear does not exclude it, but it may pick up abnormal endometrial cells. Unopposed oestrogen stimulation, either endogenous or exogenous, is associated with endometrial carcinoma. There is a 6% risk of this after five years of unopposed oral oestrogens. The addition of a progestogen reduces the incidence to a relative risk value of 0.9.

28. A C E

Maternal height is of limited value in predicting fetopelvic dispro-portion, although short mothers tend to have a higher rate of Caesarean section. Because of the large overlap in the obstetrical outcome between women with small and large dimensions the statis-tical significance of correlations between maternal height or shoe size and cephalopelvic disproportion are very limited. Non-engagement of the head may be associated with cephalopelvic disproportion in primagravidae, but it is not diagnostic. The role of X-ray pelvimetry is very limited; neither X-ray nor clinical pelvimetry have been shown to predict cephalopelvic disproportion with sufficient accuracy to justify elective Caesarean section for cephalic presentation. Cephalopelvic disproportion is best diagnosed by carefully monitored trial of labour, and X-ray pelvimetry should seldom, if ever, be necessary.

29. B C

Polyhydramnios (increased liquor volume) is associated with failure of reabsorption of liquor or an increase in production. This occurs in oesophageal atresia and open neural tube defects. Ovarian hyper-stimulation syndrome causes ascites, but not polyhydramnios. Potter's syndrome is associated with renal agenesis and this leads to oligo-rather than polyhydramnios.

30. D

Preterm or premature birth is defined by the WHO as delivery of an infant before 37 completed weeks of gestation. There is no set lower limit. It occurs in about 5–10% of births.

Causes of preterm births include:

- Unexplained 30%
  (risk factors include:
  low socioeconomic group and
  previous preterm labour)
- Genital tract infection
- Preterm premature rupture of membranes
- Multiple pregnancy (30%)
- Antepartum haemorrhage
- Cervical incompetence
- Congenital uterine abnormalities
- Elective   Intrauterine growth retardation
                   Congenital abnormalities
                   Medical disorders

About 70% of preterm labours progress to delivery.

31. D E

Bacterial vaginosis is associated with the following complications of pregnancy:

- Low birth weight
- Preterm labour
- Preterm birth
- Premature rupture of membranes
- Late miscarriage
- Chorioamnionitis
- Endometritis after Caesarean section

There is evidence that treating women with anti-anaerobic treatment may reduce chances of further premature delivery.

32. C D E

At booking it is important that the individual woman is assessed. Risks and needs need to be addressed and the antenatal care should be adapted to their own particular requirements. Seat belts must be worn in the correct fashion. As part of the full risk assessment, the body mass index should be calculated. Women need to then be offered advice about sensible weight reduction including diet and exercise and referral to a dietitian where appropriate.

A full psychiatric history is important. The term postnatal depression should only be used to describe a non psychotic depressive illness of mild to moderate severity with its onset following delivery. Read 'Why Mothers Die 1997–1999'.

33. B C

The effectiveness of advice given during pregnancy has to be questioned and evaluated as rigorously as any other intervention carried out in medicine and pregnancy. Much conflicting advice occurs about sexual activity. From assessing the evidence, it does appear that the prevention of sexual activity during pregnancy is wholly inappropriate. The evidence that maternal smoking reduces birth weight is strong, as is the evidence that excessive alcohol consumption causes damage. Excessive alcohol consumption is associated with fetal growth retardation, mental retardation and altered neonatal behaviour. There does not appear to be any scientific evidence to support decreasing work, indeed, stopping work may actually increase the amount of housework that one does and also put a stress on the financial status of the couple. Folic acid in a dose of 0.4 mg a day is now advised with 5 mg a day advised for patients who have already had a baby with spina bifida. The folic acid supplements should start three months preconception and continue until 12 weeks' gestation.

34. B C E

The most common bacteria involved are *Chlamydia trachomatis* and *Neisseria gonorrhoeae*. These cause damage to the epithelial surface and then opportunist organisms, including *Mycoplasma hominis* and anaerobes, invade.

There is high morbidity with pelvic inflammatory disease including:

20% become infertile
20% develop chronic pelvic pain
10% of those who conceive have an ectopic pregnancy.

Factors associated with pelvic inflammatory disease mirror those for sexually transmitted infections including:

- Young age
- Reduced socioeconomic influences
- African/Afro-Caribbean ethnicity
- Lower educational attainment
- Recent ascending infection

35. D E

Understanding the physiological anaemia of pregnancy is important and there is evidence that what appears to be a low haemoglobin may be beneficial in pregnancy. Very few randomised trials have monitored the effects of giving iron supplementation as a matter of routine, but it does not have any benefit on the prevention of proteinuria, hypertension, antepartum haemorrhage, or maternal infection. Anaemia may actually be detrimental to the outcome of pregnancy as a few well-conducted trials have shown that preterm delivery and low birth weight are increased. The associated pathology may be increased blood viscosity following the iron-induced macrocytosis and thus an impedance to utero-placental blood flow.

36. A C D

Ovarian hyperstimulation syndrome (OHSS) is an iatrogenic potentially life-threatening condition resulting from an excessive ovarian induction therapy. The pathophysiology of this syndrome is not clearly understood. The treatment of OHSS is often careful observation (mild or moderate OHSS). Some patients (severe OHSS) require hospitalisation and supportive therapy. In mild OHSS, the patient may complain of mild abdominal discomfort and the ovaries are usually less than 5 cm in diameter. Moderate OHSS results in more noticeable pain and vomiting, the ovaries measure between 5 and 10 cm. In the severe form, the ovaries are > 10 cm in diameter. Severe OHSS is characterised by the presence of free intraperitoneal fluid, pleural effusions, hypotension and oliguria. If no pregnancy occurs, the syndrome will typically resolve within one week. In the setting of a maintained pregnancy, slow resolution of symptoms usually occurs over one to two months. The incidence of mild and moderate forms of OHSS has been reported as between 10 and 20% of all females undergoing ovulation induction treatment and the use of gonadotrophins. Severe forms of OHSS occur in < 1% of patients undergoing ovulation induction.

37. A D

The postnatal blues are a brief period of emotional distress which can occur between the third and the tenth day postpartum. This condition is very common and occurs in 50–80% of all women who give birth. The blues are characterised by tearfulness, irritability and distress.

Postnatal psychosis is a rare and more dramatic disorder that affects 0.2% of women in the postpartum period. Symptoms may occur within the first six weeks after delivery and include: a marked disturbance in mood characterised by a very high or elated mood; or a very low, depressed mood and a disturbance in perception in which auditory or visual hallucinations can occur and behaviour disturbances.

A woman suffering from postpartum psychosis is very much at risk, and her infant and other children may also be in danger. The patient must be referred to a psychiatrist immediately.

If patient develops postnatal psychosis she has a one-in-five chance of developing it again in the next pregnancy.

38. D

The normal fetal heart rate (FHR) pattern is characterised by a baseline frequency between 110 and 150 beats per minute, presence of periodic accelerations, a normal heart rate variability between 5 and 25 beats per minute and the absence of decelerations.

Recording speeds vary from 1–3 cm per minute. Betamimetics, such as ritodrine, increase the baseline FHR and are associated with a decrease in FHR variability. Magnesium sulphate causes a decrease in FHR variability. Most cases of cerebral palsy have antecedents in the antenatal period, with only about 10% of cases having an intrapartum cause.

39. A C E

The menopause is the permanent cessation of menstruation resulting from loss of ovarian follicular activity. Natural menopause is recognised to have occurred after 12 consecutive months of amenorrhoea for which there is no obvious pathological or physiological cause. Menopause occurs with the final period and is only known with certainty in retrospect. Premature menopause is defined as menopause that occurs at an age less than two standard deviations below the mean for the reference population. In the developed world this is counted as 40 years.

40. None Correct

It is interesting that the amount of blood loss that a woman complains of can be modified by many factors, including emotional upset, marital problems, or even a fear of genital cancer. It is important to take a good history and it is true to say that, although a history may be unreliable, most women would not generally wish to have a gynaecological examination without good reason and, thus, it must commonly be assumed to be a real complaint. Clip sterilisations are not associated with heavy periods. Before rushing into a major surgical procedure, medical treatment and even more minor surgical procedures would be the first line of treatment. Abnormal menstrual bleeding may be ovulatory or anovulatory. As a rule of thumb, irregular, prolonged cycles are associated with anovulation and regular cycles are associated with ovulation and structural deformities. Anovulation is more common around puberty and the climacteric and about 20% of women who present with menstrual dysfunction will have anovulatory cycles.

41. C

There is no evidence that maternal growth hormone positively influences birth weight. Primiparity and social class are not consistently related to birth weight.

42. All True

Lie is defined as the relationship of the fetus to the long axis of mother. Cephalic presentation is the commonest presentation at term (95%). This is because of the shape of the uterine cavity which allows more room for the lower limb activities in the fundal region. Any condition that alters the shape and the position of the uterus will increase the incidence of malpresentations of the fetus, and increase the likelihood of unstable lie. These include multi-gravid uterus, polyhydramnios, prematurity, placenta praevia, fibroid, ovarian tumour in pouch of Douglas, uterine abnormalities (bicornate uterus) and fetal abnormalities such as hydrocephalus.

43. B D E

A hysterosalpingogram demonstrates tubal patency, which is subtly different from tubal function. It has a role in detecting uterine adhesions (Asherman's syndrome). It is important in the management of infertility to make sure that the investigation itself does not cause problems. A high vaginal swab as well as an endocervical swab looking for *Chlamydia* is ideal management. Giving prophylactic antibiotics should also be considered. Fibroids can impinge on the cavity, increasing the risk of failure to implant, and the role of the hysteroscope is taking over from the hysterosalpingogram.

44. A D

Bilateral salpingo-oophorectomy in premenopausal women is associated with a surgical menopause, therefore, unless it is contraindicated, hormone replacement therapy is essential. This need not be given with progestogens as there is no endometrium and unopposed oestrogens could be given orally, by implant or by patch. Premenstrual syndrome is associated with ovulation and perhaps should be called ovarian cycle syndrome. It is, therefore, eliminated by bilateral salphingo-oophorectomy at the time of a hysterectomy. The technique of an oophorectomy is not usually technically more difficult than a hysterectomy unless, of course, the ovaries are buried in adhesions. In women between the age of 45–50 it is usually advised to have the ovaries removed to decrease the risk not only of benign ovarian cysts and ovarian carcinoma but also of deep dyspareunia.

45. B

Uncomplicated vulvovaginal candidiasis affects about 75% of women at least once in their lifetime and is self-limiting. Recurrent thrush occurs in about 5% of healthy women of reproductive age.

Candida albicans has been reported to cause 75–80% of vulvovaginal candidiasis. There has been an increase in the number of cases caused by *Candida glabrata* and *Candida tropicalis*.

Well-known aetiological factors include:

- Antibiotics
- Sexual intercourse
- Diabetes mellitus

- Immunosuppression
- Pregnancy
- Combined oral contraceptive pill with high dose of oestrogen
- Hormone replacement therapy
- Intrauterine contraceptive devices.

Bubble bath, wearing non-cotton underwear and vaginal douching are largely anecdotal causes of vulvovaginal candidiasis and their causative role remains unproven.

Vaginal pH is usually normal (pH 3.5–4.5). If the pH is elevated a diagnosis of trichomoniasis or bacterial vaginosis should be considered.

46. B C D E

Dysmenorrhoea (ie painful menstruation) may be primary or secondary and is a distinctly different problem from premenstrual syndrome. Primary dysmenorrhoea occurs in young women with the onset of the ovulation cycle and without any specific underlying pathology. Abnormal levels of prostaglandins cause excessive uterine contractions. The pill is a useful form of treatment. Secondary dysmenorrhoea occurs in older women and results from underlying pelvic pathology, such as endometriosis, intrauterine contraceptive device, chronic pelvic inflammatory disease, or fibroids.

47. A B C E

Monozygotic twins occur at a rate of about 1:260 and this rate is constant with no known predisposing factors. The incidence of di-zygotic twins is influenced by:

- Race – Nigerians have a risk of about 1:20 per birth, whereas the risk in Europeans is about 1:80.
- Inheritance – a family history of twins on the mother's side is still closely associated with increased risk of twinning.
- Both increasing maternal age and parity are associated with a twin pregnancy.
- Induction of ovulation – not only does clomiphene and the use of gonadotrophins increase the risk of twins, but in vitro fertilisation is associated with an increased risk of twins. The Human Fertilisation and Embryology Authority directs that two embryos should be transferred, three in exceptional circumstances and this has reduced the twinning rates.

Complications of twinning are many and are basically associated with increased risk of all of the medical problems in pregnancy. Because of the increase in placental size there is also a risk of placenta praevia.

48. A C

In vitro fertilisation and ovum donation do not require patent tubes because the embryo is transferred back directly into the uterine cavity. The other methods require patent tubes in order to allow fertilisation to take place.

49. A C D

All types of intrauterine contraceptive device lead to an increase in the number of leukocytes, not only in the endometrium but also in the uterine and tubal fluids. Inert and copper devices lead to an increase in the levels of many prostaglandins. Copper enhances this foreign body reaction and leads to a range of biochemical changes in the endometrium affecting the enzyme system and hormone receptors. These copper ions are toxic to the sperm and blastocyst. Progestogen-releasing coils are now becoming more popular and are also useful in heavy periods. Inert devices are no longer available in the United Kingdom. As the surface area of the inert device is reduced so the side-effects of bleeding and pain are minimised but the failure rate increases. With the introduction of copper, one can use a smaller device without this loss of efficiency. The levonorgestrel device reduces menstrual blood flow, but the copper-containing devices do not. The intrauterine contraceptive device is a highly effective method which is nearly always reversible with no known unwanted systemic side-effects. It is independent of intercourse and does not require much motivation nor day-to-day action. It is relatively cheap, easy to distribute and does not affect the postpartum mother.

50. C E

From mid-pregnancy onwards the fetal kidney contributes increasingly to amniotic fluid volume, contributing some 500 ml per day by term; in renal agenesis the liquor volume is greatly reduced. The volume of amniotic fluid may be estimated by ultrasound, but not accurately. Liquor volumes are higher than average in rhesus-affected pregnancies and grossly increased in hydrops fetalis. Amniocentesis may permit amniotic fluid to leak away, thus reducing the volume. Pre-eclampsia and intrauterine growth retardation are both associated with reduced amniotic fluid volumes.

51. B D E

In a menstruating woman if the combined oral contraceptive pill is started on day one then extra precautions are not required for seven days. If the combined oral contraceptive pill is started on day three or later extra precautions are required for seven days. If women are postpartum and not lactating then the combined oral contraceptive pill can be started on day 21 when there is a low risk of thrombosis. As first ovulation has been reported by day 28 extra precautions are not needed if started on day 21. During lactation the combined oral contraceptive pill is not recommended. Progestogen-only injectables are preferred. After induced early abortion or miscarriage the combined oral contraceptive pill can be started the same or next day to avoid postoperative vomiting. Extra precautions are not needed for seven days.

52. A C D

Cephalohaematoma is caused by bleeding that occurs below the periosteum and is associated with a ventouse delivery. Sometimes the swelling takes a long time to resolve and may actually lead to a calcified ridge. The resolution can be associated with an increased jaundice level. Physiological jaundice occurs between days two and five. Owing to the immaturity of the liver enzymes, there is a raised level of unconjugated bilirubin. Infection may lead to jaundice and it is therefore important to investigate these babies. Full blood count, blood cultures, lumbar puncture, chest X-ray and midstream urine specimen are important. If rhesus incompatibility is suspected, then full investigations include:

- Coombs' test
- Maternal blood group
- Infant blood group
- The detection of anti-A or anti-B haemolysins in the maternal circulation.

Hypothyroidism is associated with jaundice, but this is a prolonged jaundice.

53. C

The dangers of hypoxia and fetal trauma are greater in the flexed/footling types. Meconium often reflects pressure on the fetal abdomen and is not a reliable sign of distress. Variable fetal heart rate decelerations are commonly due to cord compression. Elective caesarean section, in many units, is the preferred mode of delivery. The obstetric forceps enable a safe delivery of the aftercoming head, by ensuring the head is not delivered too slowly, resulting in cerebral hypoxia, nor too rapidly, which may cause intracranial haemorrhage.

54. A B C

It is very important to learn the common side-effects of drugs. Oestrogen is often associated with weight gain, although studies have not always confirmed this. Acyclovir, which is the treatment of herpes simplex and varicella zoster, can cause a rash and gastrointestinal disturbances as well as rises in bilirubin and liver enzymes. It can also increase blood urea and creatinine as well as cause headache, fatigue and neurological reactions, including dizziness. Fluconazole, used in the treatment of thrush, can cause not only nausea, abdominal discomfort, diarrhoea and flatulence but occasionally can cause abnormalities of the liver enzymes. Bromocriptine can cause nausea, vomiting, constipation, headaches, dizziness and postural hypotension. In particular, vasospasm in fingers can occur in patients with Raynaud's syndrome. Danazol has an androgenic effect and is therefore associated with reduction in breast size as well as acne, oily skin and possible hirsutism.

55. B C E
Obesity is a risk factor for hypertension, but not for pre-eclampsia. Women who have had hypertension on the combined oral contraceptive pill are at risk, as are those with autoimmune disorders.

56. B C
Increasing maternal age increases the incidence of a hydatidiform mole. Surgical evacuation with human chorionic gonadotrophin follow-up is the treatment of choice. Choriocarcinoma is treated by methotrexate and other chemotherapeutic agents.

57. A B E
The signs and symptoms of ovarian cancer have been described as vague or silent; around 10% of ovarian cancer is diagnosed in the early stages. Symptoms typically occur in advanced stages. Symptoms may include any of the following: loss of appetite, nausea and a bloated feeling, unexplained weight gain, abdominal distension, abnormal vaginal bleeding, and changes in bowel or bladder habits. Most of the ovarian tumours are of epithelial origin. These are rare before the age of 35. The incidence increases with age and the peak in the 50–70 year age group. CA125 is a tumour marker for ovarian cancer. About half the women who have early-stage ovarian cancer do not have raised levels of CA125. Also, it can be raised in a variety of other conditions, such as endometriosis, fibroids, pelvic inflammatory disease, or even pregnancy.

58. All True
This Report has evaluated other factors which contribute to increased maternal mortality. Women from low socioeconomic classes (risk of

death is 20 times higher than in women from high social class), young women under 18 years of age and women from ethnic minority groups (twice as likely to die as white women) had higher mortality rates than among the population as a whole. Also, the report has shown high mortality rate among women from the traditional travelling community and women with late antenatal booking (after 24 weeks). Other factors were also associated with an increased risk of death; such as increasing maternal age and increasing parity. Many women in this Enquiry were also obese. **The Confidential Enquiries into Maternal Deaths in the United Kingdom (1997–1999), Executive Summary and Key Recommendations, RCOG website.**

59. B C D E

The highest incidence of damage is 50% at four weeks. The risk decreases after the first trimester. Gammaglobulin, if given, may be protective.

60. A B C E

Uterovaginal prolapse results from weakness of the pelvic support, including muscles, ligaments and fascia. Multiparity, long labour, instrumental deliveries and vaginal delivery of large babies are some of the factors that predispose a woman to developing uterine prolapse. Menopause can weaken the pelvic floor because of diminished oestrogen levels. Increased intra-abdominal pressure on a long-term basis can contribute to genital prolapse, for example, heavy lifting, obesity, ascites, chronic coughing and chronic constipation are also important contributing factors in genital prolapse. No relation has been found between uterovaginal prolapse and LLETZ.

MCQ Practice Exam 2

60 Questions: time allowed 2 hours. Indicate your answers clearly by putting a tick or cross against each answer option.

1. **There is a recognisable chromosome abnormality in the following:**

   ☐ **A** Klinefelter's syndrome
   ☐ **B** Tay–Sachs disease
   ☐ **C** Achondroplasia
   ☐ **D** Cri-du-chat syndrome
   ☐ **E** Patau's syndrome

2. **Endometriosis can be treated by**

   ☐ **A** medroxyprogesterone acetate
   ☐ **B** danazol
   ☐ **C** evening primrose oil
   ☐ **D** mefenamic acid
   ☐ **E** luteinising hormone releasing hormone analogues

3. **An oblique lie**

   ☐ **A** may be transitory
   ☐ **B** usually turns to a longitudinal lie
   ☐ **C** after 33 weeks needs to be admitted to hospital due to the risk of cord prolapse
   ☐ **D** should be treated by external cephalic version (ECV) at 37 weeks
   ☐ **E** is associated with placenta praevia

4. **The following statements about breech presentation are true:**

   ☐ **A** At 28 weeks the incidence of breech presentation is 40%
   ☐ **B** The incidence of breech presentation at term is 3–4%
   ☐ **C** The perinatal mortality and morbidity with breech presentations is the same as with vertex
   ☐ **D** All women with uncomplicated breech pregnancy at term (37–42 weeks) should be offered external cephalic version
   ☐ **E** The best method of delivering a term frank or complete breech singleton is by planned Caesarean section

5. **The following renal changes are typical of normal pregnancy:**

   ☐ **A** Increased glomerular filtration rate
   ☐ **B** Decreased excretion of urate
   ☐ **C** Increased excretion of folate
   ☐ **D** Increased excretion of glucose
   ☐ **E** Ureteric dilatation

6. **Pruritus vulvae may be associated with**

   ☐ **A** diabetes
   ☐ **B** Raynaud's disease
   ☐ **C** threadworm
   ☐ **D** thyroid disease
   ☐ **E** renal failure

7. **Pregnancy is associated with**

   ☐ **A** an increase in cardiac output
   ☐ **B** a decrease in central venous pressure
   ☐ **C** an increase in peripheral resistance
   ☐ **D** an increase in pulse rate
   ☐ **E** a decrease in stroke volume

8. **Depo-Provera**

   ☐ **A** is the most widely used form of injectable contraception
   ☐ **B** can effect lactation
   ☐ **C** has a failure rate ranging from 5 to 7 pregnancies per 100 women years
   ☐ **D** in adequate doses suppresses ovulation
   ☐ **E** has no effect on cervical mucus

9. **The following definitions are correct:**

   ☐ **A** A late death is a death occurring between 42 days and one year after abortion or delivery that is due to direct or indirect maternal causes
   ☐ **B** A stillbirth is the birth, after 24 weeks' gestation, of an infant that does not show signs of life
   ☐ **C** Perinatal mortality is defined as stillbirths plus first-week neonatal deaths expressed per thousand total births
   ☐ **D** Neonatal death is a live-born infant who dies within 28 days of birth (whatever gestation if signs of life are noted)
   ☐ **E** Maternities is a count of the number of mothers delivered of live or stillborn infants as distinct from the number of babies born which includes twins and other multiple births

10. Endometriosis

- ☐ **A** occurs with increasing age
- ☐ **B** has a peak incidence between the ages of 50 and 55
- ☐ **C** occurs in about 1% of Caucasians
- ☐ **D** the extent of the disease correlates well with the symptoms
- ☐ **E** may be a normal clinical finding

11. Nonsensitised rhesus (Rh)-negative women should receive anti-D immunoglobulin in the following situations:

- ☐ **A** Ectopic pregnancy after 12 weeks
- ☐ **B** Any miscarriage after eight weeks
- ☐ **C** All miscarriages in which surgical evacuation is performed
- ☐ **D** All miscarriages in which medical evacuation is performed
- ☐ **E** Any threatened miscarriage when there is heavy vaginal bleeding or associated abdominal pain

12. Medical treatment of dysfunctional uterine bleeding includes

- ☐ **A** oral contraceptive
- ☐ **B** mefenamic acid
- ☐ **C** cyclical progestogens
- ☐ **D** transcervical resection of the endometrium
- ☐ **E** evening primrose oil

13. The following statements are true regarding cervical smears:

- ☐ **A** A negative result excludes frank carcinoma
- ☐ **B** Persistent inflammatory results warrant colposcopic examination
- ☐ **C** Koilocytosis is suggestive of human papillomavirus (HPV)
- ☐ **D** Dyskaryosis is caused by *Trichomonas vaginalis*
- ☐ **E** They are best performed postnatally at six weeks

14. Management of a pregnant woman who presents with chickenpox includes:

- ☐ **A** Isolation from all other pregnant women and neonates
- ☐ **B** Delivery ideally should be delayed until 5–7 days after the onset of maternal illness
- ☐ **C** If delivery occurs within five days of maternal infection, then the neonate should be given varicella zoster immunoglobulin (VZIG) as soon as possible
- ☐ **D** Varicella pneumonia is an indication for treatment with intravenous acyclovir
- ☐ **E** Where maternal infection occurs five days before or two days after delivery there is a 20–30% risk of varicella of the newborn

45

15. The following statements about miscarriage are true:

- ☐ **A** Miscarriage is known to occur in 3% of clinical pregnancies
- ☐ **B** In a threatened miscarriage bed-rest should be encouraged
- ☐ **C** Medical management is not an acceptable method in the management of confirmed miscarriage
- ☐ **D** Risks of surgical evacuation include intra-abdominal trauma
- ☐ **E** If a woman is undergoing surgical evacuation she should be screened for *Chlamydia trachomatis*

16. The following statements about the gestational age of a newborn baby are true:

- ☐ **A** at 36 weeks of age the ear returns to its shape after folding
- ☐ **B** at 38 weeks of age there is no palpable breast tissue
- ☐ **C** at 38 weeks of age the testes have few scrotal rugae
- ☐ **D** at 40 weeks of age there is good arm recoil after extension at the elbow
- ☐ **E** at 40 weeks of age the baby is pale pink with slight superficial skin peeling

17. The following statements about placenta praevia are true:

- ☐ **A** Transvaginal ultrasound is safe in the presence of placenta praevia
- ☐ **B** Patients with major placenta praevia, with recent evidence, do not need to be admitted to hospital
- ☐ **C** Cervical cerclage should be considered
- ☐ **D** Caesarean section is the management of choice for women whose placenta is 10 cm or less from the os
- ☐ **E** A hysterectomy may be required to help control haemorrhage at the time of Caesarean section

18. Endometriosis:

- ☐ **A** Occurs in about 20% of women being investigated for infertility
- ☐ **B** May present with a pelvic mass
- ☐ **C** Can be easily diagnosed by ultrasound scanning
- ☐ **D** May be associated with a raised CA125
- ☐ **E** Is always symptomatic

19. Neonatal hypocalcaemia

- [ ] **A** may be due to maternal dietary deficiency
- [ ] **B** often accompanies hypoglycaemia
- [ ] **C** may cause permanent brain damage
- [ ] **D** is a common cause of convulsions
- [ ] **E** is seen in association with a normal maternal blood calcium concentration

20. Polycystic ovarian syndrome (PCOS)

- [ ] **A** was first described by Stein and Leventhal in 1935
- [ ] **B** is associated with a low serum luteinising hormone level
- [ ] **C** may be associated with anovulation, hirsutism, obesity and reduced ovarian stroma
- [ ] **D** can be associated with hypoinsulinaemia
- [ ] **E** may be associated with recurrent miscarriages

21. Concerning carcinoma of the cervix

- [ ] **A** it is the commonest malignant cause of female deaths
- [ ] **B** the death rate has been significantly reduced by the British screening programme
- [ ] **C** the majority of women dying from the condition have never had a smear
- [ ] **D** it has a decreased incidence in smokers
- [ ] **E** the treatment of choice is radiotherapy in the obese woman

22. The following statements about hormone replacement therapy used in specific medical conditions are true:

- [ ] **A** There is significant risk of increasing the size of a fibroid
- [ ] **B** HRT is contraindicated in diabetes mellitus
- [ ] **C** HRT is contraindicated in otosclerosis
- [ ] **D** HRT should be considered in renal failure
- [ ] **E** HRT may increase the risk of gall bladder disease

23. In Down's syndrome

- ☐ **A** most patients have an extra number 21 chromosome
- ☐ **B** trisomy is usually due to non-disjunction during meiosis
- ☐ **C** a female with Down's syndrome would never have a normal child
- ☐ **D** women over the age of 40 years have a risk of 1 in 200 of having a child with Down's syndrome
- ☐ **E** an affected fetus may be associated with a reduced serum α-fetoprotein concentration in amniotic fluid

24. The following micro-organisms are capable of penetrating the placental barrier and infecting the fetus:

- ☐ **A** *Staphylococcus aureus*
- ☐ **B** *Toxoplasma gondii*
- ☐ **C** cytomegalovirus
- ☐ **D** varicella zoster virus
- ☐ **E** hepatitis B virus

25. Scabies

- ☐ **A** is due to infestation by the mite *Sarcoptes scabiei*
- ☐ **B** infestation is after close physical contact
- ☐ **C** symptoms usually occur within 12 hours of infestation
- ☐ **D** treatment is by the application of 25% benzyl benzoate
- ☐ **E** itching is usually relieved within 48 hours after successful treatment

26. Gestational diabetes

- ☐ **A** is defined as glucose intolerance appearing during pregnancy
- ☐ **B** is associated with a small increase in perinatal mortality
- ☐ **C** is best treated with insulin
- ☐ **D** is associated with fetal macrosomia
- ☐ **E** if treated with insulin, reduces the incidence of fetal macrosomia

27. Luteinising hormone releasing hormone (LHRH) analogues are effective in the treatment of

- ☐ **A** menorrhagia
- ☐ **B** endometriosis
- ☐ **C** uterine fibroids
- ☐ **D** osteoporosis
- ☐ **E** granuloma cell tumour of the ovary

28. In the fetus

- ☐ **A** the umbilical arteries carry oxygenated blood
- ☐ **B** the ductus venosus short circuits the capillaries of the liver
- ☐ **C** the right atrium contains a mixture of oxygenated and venous blood
- ☐ **D** the foramen ovale connects the ventricles of the heart
- ☐ **E** the ductus arteriosus joins the aorta proximal to the aortic arch

29. Respiratory distress syndrome of the newborn

- ☐ **A** is always obvious at birth when present
- ☐ **B** causes pathognomonic changes on the chest X-ray
- ☐ **C** is unusual in full-term babies
- ☐ **D** responds to supplementation of lung surfactants
- ☐ **E** should be treated routinely with antibiotics

30. The following treatments for hyperemesis are evidence based:

- ☐ **A** Antihistamines
- ☐ **B** Corticosteroids
- ☐ **C** Phenothiazines
- ☐ **D** Dietary ginger
- ☐ **E** Acupressure

31. Genital warts

- ☐ **A** are benign mesodermal growths on the external perianal and perigenital region
- ☐ **B** caused by the herpes simplex virus
- ☐ **C** are sexually transmitted
- ☐ **D** may resolve spontaneously
- ☐ **E** progress to cancer in 3% of cases

32. Vulvodynia

- ☐ **A** is a term used to describe a specific type of vulval pain characterised by burning, stinging, irritation and rawness
- ☐ **B** may be caused by vulval eczema
- ☐ **C** can cause dyspareunia
- ☐ **D** may be caused by allergy
- ☐ **E** can be treated with local corticosteroids

33. **The following methods can be used to screen for genetic disease during pregnancy:**

☐ **A** Ultrasound
☐ **B** Amniocentesis
☐ **C** Chorionic villus sampling
☐ **D** X-ray
☐ **E** A combination of α-fetoprotein, β human chorionic gonadotrophin and oestriol levels

34. **Pelvic inflammatory disease**

☐ **A** is inflammation of the upper genital tract in women typically involving the Fallopian tubes, ovaries and surrounding structures
☐ **B** is best diagnosed by clinical symptoms and signs
☐ **C** is always symptomatic
☐ **D** in most cases is due to an ascending infection from the cervix
☐ **E** can be prevented by vaginal douching

35. **The following are useful tests for the assessment of fetal wellbeing in the third trimester:**

☐ **A** vaginal ultrasound measurement of crown–rump length
☐ **B** human placental lactogen measurement
☐ **C** serum α-fetoprotein
☐ **D** fetal movement counting
☐ **E** amniotic fluid volume measurement

36. **Women with heart disease in pregnancy**

☐ **A** with good multidisciplinary care are at no greater risk of maternal death
☐ **B** can be given oxytocin in the usual way
☐ **C** can present with pyrexia of unknown origin
☐ **D** are at additional risk if they have a pulmonary vascular disease
☐ **E** should be given careful pre-pregnancy counselling

37. **Breast-fed children are less likely to have the following:**

☐ **A** Ear infections (otitis media)
☐ **B** Allergies
☐ **C** Vomiting
☐ **D** Diarrhoea
☐ **E** Pneumonia, wheezing and bronchiolitis

38. Oblique lie is associated with

- ☐ **A** multiparity
- ☐ **B** uterine abnormalities
- ☐ **C** fundal placenta
- ☐ **D** pelvic tumours
- ☐ **E** small pelvic inlet

39. With regard to the menopause:

- ☐ **A** Age of the menopause may be determined *in utero*
- ☐ **B** It occurs earlier in women with Down's syndrome
- ☐ **C** It occurs later in smokers
- ☐ **D** Japanese race/ethnicity may be associated with later age of natural menopause
- ☐ **E** It results in a fall of oestrogen production

40. Ovarian hyperstimulation syndrome

- ☐ **A** is a complication of induction of ovulation
- ☐ **B** usually occurs after human chorionic gonadotrophin has been given
- ☐ **C** is associated with polycystic ovarian syndrome
- ☐ **D** is associated with a predisposition to thrombosis
- ☐ **E** can be fatal

41. Heartburn in pregnancy

- ☐ **A** affects about two-thirds of all women at some stage during pregnancy
- ☐ **B** is commonly associated with eating or lying down
- ☐ **C** can be treated effectively with diazepam
- ☐ **D** magnesium salts would appear to be one of the safest treatment options
- ☐ **E** may be treated with dilute hydrochloric acid

42. Fetal biophysical profile scoring

- ☐ **A** has resulted in the birth of babies with lower Apgar scores
- ☐ **B** has resulted in a reduction in the perinatal mortality rate
- ☐ **C** includes serum oestradiol measurement
- ☐ **D** includes fetal tone measurement on ultrasound scan
- ☐ **E** includes fetal breathing assessment

43. The following conditions are thought to be commonly caused by viruses:

- [ ] **A** Condyloma acuminatum
- [ ] **B** Bartholinitis
- [ ] **C** Cervical intra-epithelial neoplasia
- [ ] **D** Lichen sclerosus
- [ ] **E** Acute vulval ulcers

44. Cervical cancer:

- [ ] **A** Human papillomavirus infection is a major risk factor for development of pre-invasive or invasive carcinoma of the cervix
- [ ] **B** Cervical cancer can be presented as postmenopausal bleeding
- [ ] **C** The incidence of cervical carcinoma is 9.3 cases per 10 000 women
- [ ] **D** The UK has the highest recorded incidence in the European Union
- [ ] **E** Deaths from cervical cancer have fallen by more than 40%

45. A low haemoglobin in pregnancy

- [ ] **A** should initially be treated with iron
- [ ] **B** depends on a complex relation between red cell mass and plasma volume
- [ ] **C** is usually associated with an iron deficiency anaemia
- [ ] **D** can be improved more quickly with the addition of ascorbic acid
- [ ] **E** if associated with a megaloblastic anaemia in pregnancy is almost always due to folate deficiency

46. Treatment of benign hirsutism includes

- [ ] **A** the oral contraceptive pill
- [ ] **B** danazol
- [ ] **C** cyproterone acetate
- [ ] **D** prednisolone
- [ ] **E** electrolysis

47. The following statements about perimenopausal contraception are true:

- [ ] A Measurement of the oestradiol levels are a valid method of identifying the menopause
- [ ] B It is accepted practice that contraception is required for a further one year when the menopause occurs in women over the age of 50 years
- [ ] C It is accepted practice that contraception is required for a further two years when the menopause occurs in women under the age of 50 years
- [ ] D Hormone replacement therapy with progestogens is a reliable form of contraceptive
- [ ] E Follicle-stimulating hormone levels are reliable in women taking the progestogen-only pill as this does not affect testing

48. Vulval carcinoma

- [ ] A is associated with pruritus vulvae
- [ ] B is usually multifocal
- [ ] C is uncommon in African patients
- [ ] D is more common in multiparous patients
- [ ] E is best treated by chemotherapy

49. Polyhydramnios may be associated with

- [ ] A abruptio placentae
- [ ] B intrauterine growth retardation
- [ ] C fetal oesophageal atresia
- [ ] D preterm labour
- [ ] E postpartum haemorrhage

50. A progestogen

- [ ] A causes a withdrawal bleed on an oestrogen-primed endometrium
- [ ] B can be used as a screening test for endometrial hyperplasia
- [ ] C is the treatment of choice for menorrhagia
- [ ] D when given to a postmenopausal woman can cause a decrease in the incidence of endometrial carcinoma
- [ ] E should be given routinely to all postmenopausal women who are on oestrogen therapy

51. Regarding gynaecological malignancies

- [ ] **A** endometrial carcinoma spreads to lymphatics less readily than cervical carcinoma
- [ ] **B** radiotherapy is the treatment of choice for a malignant pyometra
- [ ] **C** in a Wertheim's hysterectomy the lower third of the vagina is excised
- [ ] **D** the ovaries may be conserved in the surgical treatment of carcinoma of the corpus uteri
- [ ] **E** renal failure is a common cause of death in cervical carcinoma

52. The following statements about infection in pregnancy are true:

- [ ] **A** Rubella is an RNA virus
- [ ] **B** Toxoplasmosis can be treated by spiramycin
- [ ] **C** Congenital varicella syndrome occurs in about 1:1000 deliveries
- [ ] **D** *Listeria* is associated with spontaneous abortion
- [ ] **E** *Listeria* can be treated by ampicillin

53. Dilatation and curettage

- [ ] **A** was performed at a rate of 71.1 per 1000 women in 1989–1990
- [ ] **B** is being replaced by outpatient procedures
- [ ] **C** samples all the endometrium
- [ ] **D** has a 5% false-negative rate
- [ ] **E** is associated with uterine perforation

54. Treatment of acute vulvovaginal candidiasis includes:

- [ ] **A** Topical clotrimazole 1%
- [ ] **B** Topical econazole 1%
- [ ] **C** Topical miconazole 2%
- [ ] **D** Oral fluconazole 150 mg stat
- [ ] **E** Itraconazole 200 mg twice daily for one day

55. Constipation during pregnancy

☐ **A** can be treated with magnesium salts during pregnancy
☐ **B** can be treated with dioctyl sodium sulphosuccinate during pregnancy
☐ **C** can be prevented by increasing the amount of fibre in the diet
☐ **D** is associated with a decrease in gut motility
☐ **E** is particularly bad in the first trimester of pregnancy

56. During pregnancy

☐ **A** glycosuria is an effective test of carbohydrate intolerance
☐ **B** fasting plasma glucose concentration is decreased
☐ **C** fasting plasma insulin concentration is decreased
☐ **D** the oral glucose tolerance test alters with advancing gestation
☐ **E** two hours after an oral glucose load, plasma insulin concentration should have returned to fasting levels

57. An 18-year-old female complains of never having had a period. She has normal breast development and is 157 cm in height. Secondary sexual development commenced three years previously. Chromosomal analysis is normal and blood tests indicate a serum luteinising hormone of 10.6 IU/ litre, and serum follicle-stimulating hormone of 3.6 IU/litre. Possible explanations include

☐ **A** androgen insensitivity syndrome
☐ **B** polycystic ovarian disease
☐ **C** constitutional delayed puberty
☐ **D** primary ovarian failure
☐ **E** imperforate hymen

58. Common causes of meningitis in the newborn include

☐ **A** *Neisseria meningitidis*
☐ **B** *Haemophilus influenzae*
☐ **C** *Escherichia coli*
☐ **D** group B streptococci
☐ **E** pneumococci

59. Why Mothers Die 1997–1999

☐ **A** summarises recommendations made in the third Report of the Confidential Enquiries into Maternal Deaths in the UK
☐ **B** is the longest running audit in the world
☐ **C** states that women from the low socio-economic classes are five times more likely to die than women in the highest social classes
☐ **D** states that the maternal mortality rate in the UK for this triennium is 20 deaths per 100 000 maternities
☐ **E** states that the direct maternal mortality rate is 5.0 deaths per 100 000 maternities

60. Advantages of copper-containing intrauterine contraceptive devices include

☐ **A** they are effective
☐ **B** they are reversible
☐ **C** they are cheap
☐ **D** they reduce menstrual blood loss
☐ **E** there are no known unwanted systemic effects

MCQ Practice Exam 2: Answers and Teaching Notes

1. **A D E**

   Klinefelter's syndrome characteristically has an XXY chromosome complement. Cri-du-chat syndrome is due to deletion of part of the short arm of chromosome 5. Patau's syndrome displays trisomy 13. Tay–Sachs disease is associated with a single autosomal recessive gene and achondroplasia is due to an autosomal dominant gene neither of which is normally recognisable without special techniques.

2. **A B E**

   There are many different forms of medical treatment for endometriosis, but the aim is to induce either a pseudo-pregnancy or a pseudo-menopausal state. The progestogens, such as medroxyprogesterone acetate and gestrinone, are helpful. Danazol suppresses mid-cycle luteinising hormone surge and produces a high androgen gonadotrophin secretion by the pituitary. It has marked androgenic side effects and is rarely used nowadays. This low oestrogen environment does not appear to cause a significant reduction in bone density.

3. **A B E**

   An oblique lie is associated with multiparity, uterine abnormality, fundal placenta, pelvic tumours, small pelvic inlet and polyhydramnios. Due to the risk of cord prolapse, admission is recommended at or around 37 weeks' gestation.

4. **B D E**

   The incidence of breech presentation is around 20% at 28 weeks with the incidence at term being 3–4%. There is a higher perinatal mortality and morbidity with breech presentation principally due to:

   - Prematurity
   - Congenital malformation
   - Birth asphyxia
   - Birth trauma

   External cephalic version has been subjected to rigorous scientific studies. There is a significant reduction in the risk of Caesarean section in women where there is an intention to undertake external cephalic version without any increased risk to the baby.

The Term Breech Trial conducted via the Canadian MRC was stopped early because it was confirmed that vaginal delivery is more hazardous than elective Caesarean section. Perinatal death for term frank/complete breech fetus with planned Caesarean birth was reduced by 75%.

5. **A C D E**

There is an increase in the glomerular filtration rate in normal pregnancy. This leads to an increased excretion of folate and glucose. Because of the latter the renal threshold may be reached and glycosuria may appear in pregnancy. Urate excretion increases by 40%. Ureteric dilatation is known to occur, possibly due to a progesterone effect.

6. **A C D E**

The following are all causes of pruritus vulvae:

Fungal infections
- *Candida*
- tinea

Parasitic infections
- scabies
- pediculosis pubis
- threadworm

Viral infections
- herpes
- warts
- molluscum contagiosum

Sexually transmitted diseases
- trichomoniasis
- gonorrhoea

Local dermatological conditions
- contact dermatitis
- psoriasis, etc

General medical disorders
- diabetes mellitus
- thyroid disease
- liver disease
- Crohn's disease

- chronic renal failure
- polycythaemia
- chronic lymphatic leukaemia

Vulval dystrophies
- tumours
- miscellaneous, eg foreign bodies
- generalised dermatosis
- drug reactions
- psychogenic
- lichen sclerosis

7. **A D**

Our understanding of the changes in cardiac output in pregnancy has evolved gradually with changes in measurement techniques. The most widely accepted view is that in the normal pregnant woman at rest, not lying supine, cardiac output rises from early pregnancy to a peak at around 20 weeks' gestation which is approximately 5 litres/min or 40% above the nonpregnant level; this level seems to be maintained throughout the rest of pregnancy. Although venous pressure in the legs has been shown to increase during pregnancy, that in the arms is unaltered and central venous pressure is said to remain in the range 2–5 cm water. Peripheral resistance is calculated from the mean arterial pressure divided by cardiac output; since cardiac output is increased and arterial blood pressure if anything falls slightly, it follows that peripheral resistance must be decreased. The fall has been estimated at between 20 and 40% and seems to be maximal in mid-pregnancy; this is due to the opening up of new vascular beds within the uterus and placenta and a general relaxation in peripheral vascular tone. The increased cardiac output of pregnancy is achieved by both an increase in heart rate (averaging 15 bpm) and stroke volume (from 65 to 70 ml); again these changes are present from early pregnancy.

8. **A D**

Depo-Provera is the most widely used injectable method of contraceptive which is effective, reversible and does not have a deleterious effect on lactation and does not interfere with sexual activity. The failure rate ranges between 0 and 0.7 pregnancies per 100 women years. A dose of 150 mg of Depo-Provera effectively suppresses ovulation by inhibiting the secretion of the pituitary gonadotrophins. It alters the yield, composition and physical characteristics of cervical mucus.

9. A B C D E

Learn these definitions!

10. A E

If looked for at the time of laparoscopy, mild endometriosis is found in about 10% of cases. However, it may be totally asymptomatic and thus it could be counted as a 'normal' finding. The menopause, either natural or induced, will prevent the recurrence of endometriosis.

11. C D E

The following recommendations are based on the RCOG guidelines for Rh prophylaxis. Anti-D should be given to all non-sensitised Rh-negative women who:

- Miscarry after 12 weeks – whether complete or incomplete
- Those who miscarry below 12 weeks when the uterus is evacuated surgically or medically
- Threatened miscarriage after 12 weeks
- Threatened miscarriage below 12 weeks when the bleeding is heavy or there is abdominal pain.

12. A B C

Medical treatment of dysfunctional uterine bleeding does depend on the individual's medical history as well as her wishes. Progestogens have a limited role if taken orally, but the progestogen-releasing coil is an effective treatment option.

13. B C

A cervical smear may be negative in the presence of frank carcinoma. The surface of the malignant tissue is often ulcerated and the sample from the smear shows necrotic debris and possible inflammatory cells. A diagnosis of carcinoma can only be substantiated by cervical biopsy. Inflammatory smears require further investigation to exclude cervical intraepithelial neoplasia (CIN) and human papillomavirus (HPV) infection. Some studies have shown that 10% of inflammatory smears have CIN and >20% are associated with HPV. *Trichomonas vaginalis* may produce an anti-inflammatory picture, which the inexperienced cytologist may find difficult to interpret, but the cells will not be dyskaryotic. Dyskaryotic cells show abnormal nuclear changes; large nuclei with increased chromatin and evidence of mitoses. Koilocytes are cells which appear empty due to the presence of HPV within them. Cervical smears taken at the postnatal clinic at six weeks are notoriously inaccurate and are often obscured by inflammatory material from the lochia and necrotic tissue.

14. All True

15. D

Sensitive terms used to replace older terms include:

Older terms	New Terms
Spontaneous abortion	Miscarriage
Incomplete abortion	Incomplete miscarriage
Missed abortion (presence of non-viable fetus)	Silent miscarriage
Anembryonic pregnancy (absent fetal echo)	Delayed miscarriage Early fetal demise

Miscarriage occurs in about 10–20% of all clinical pregnancies accounting for about 50 000 in-patient admission to hospital in the UK annually. This figure may be reducing with the introduction of early pregnancy assessment units (EPAU) and more conservative management. Bed-rest does not change the outcome of a threatened miscarriage, it may increase the risk of deep vein thrombosis and pulmonary embolism.

Medical evacuation and expectant management are accepted alternative techniques although they have not replaced surgical evacuation. Various medical methods have been described including:

Prostaglandin analogues
– gemeprost
– misoprostol

With or without anti-progesterone priming – mifepristone

Serious risks of surgical evacuation include

- Perforation
- Cervical tears
- Intra-abdominal trauma
- Intrauterine adhesions
- Haemorrhage
- Venous thrombosis and embolism
- Infection

The routine use of antibiotic prophylaxis is reducing the incidence of pelvic infection after induced abortion has been demonstrated. It is recommended that all at-risk women undergoing surgical evacuation should be screened for *Chlamydia*.

16. A D E

See the table on pages 63–64 – estimation of gestation of newborn babies.

17. A E

Transvaginal ultrasound is safe and more accurate than trans-abdominal in locating the placenta. There have been numerous studies investigating transvaginal ultrasound for placenta praevia and none have demonstrated an increase in bleeding.

Recent guidelines from the RCOG have concluded that in-patient management is still appropriate for women with major praevia in the third trimester. There is no evidence that cervical cerclage provides any benefit. The mode of delivery should be based on clinical judgement but a placenta encroaching within 2 cm of the internal os is a contraindication to attempting vaginal delivery.

Excessive life-threatening bleeding can occur at the time of Caesarean section. Techniques to control bleeding include:

- Uterotonic agents
- Bimanual compression
- Aortic compression
- 'B-Lynch' sutures
- Internal iliac artery ligation
- Hysterectomy

18. A B D

The prevalence of endometriosis in the following conditions is:

- Women being investigated for infertility – 20%
- Women undergoing sterilisation – 6%
- Women being investigated for chronic abdominal pain – 15%
- Women undergoing hysterectomy – 25%

The following can be used for diagnosis:

Symptoms: Dysmenorrhoea
Pelvic pain
Infertility
Secondary dysmenorrhoea
Deep dyspareunia
Pelvic pain

ESTIMATION OF GESTATION OF NEWBORN BABIES

Week of gestation	Colour & texture of skin	Ear firmness and cartilage response to folding	Diameter of palpable breast tissue	Male external genitalia
28	Uniformly red Smooth, thin 'transparent'	No resistance to folding Stays folded		Testes not palpable
30			Not palpable	Testes palpable above scrotum Few scrotal rugae
32		Very pliable but does not quite stay folded		
34	Pink, not completely smooth		Nodule 2 mm	
36		Returns after folding; Cartilage palpable at edge of pinna	Nodule 4 mm	Testes in scrotum Obvious scrotal rugae
38	Pale pink, varying; Slight superficial peeling	Springs back rapidly Cartilage palpable throughout		
40	Pink, thick with widespread peeling		Nodule 7 mm or more	
42				

ESTIMATION OF GESTATION OF NEWBORN BABIES

Week of gestation	Female external genitalia	'Scarf sign'	Heel brought towards opposite ear	Arm recoil after extension at elbow	Dorsiflexion of foot (angle with tibial surface)
28	Labia majora widely separated labia minora very prominent ↓	↓	No resistance ↓	↓	↓
30		No resistance ↓	Slight resistance ↓	None ↓	40° ↓
32					
34		Slight resistance ↓	Heel reaches ear with difficulty ↓		
36	Labia minora nearly covered by labia majora ↓	Elbow reaches midline of body ↓		Slight ↓	20 ↓
38		Elbow reaches only to nipple line or less ↓	Impossible to get heel to ear ↓		Dorsum of foot will just touch tibial surface ↓
40	Labia minora covered by labia majora ↓			Good ↓	
42	↓	↓	↓	↓	↓

Signs: Abdominal/vaginal tenderness
Pelvic mass

[May be asymptomatic]

Investigations: Laparoscopy is Gold Standard
Transvaginal scan – of limited value
MRI scan – of limited value
CA125 – may be raised and may help to diagnosis or
monitor disease progress.

19. B D E

Calcium is actively transported across the placenta to the fetus against a concentration gradient. Soon after birth the serum calcium concentration in the baby falls, maximally on the second day. Thereafter the level rises towards adult values during the next 2–3 days. It is therefore largely unrelated to maternal blood calcium at or around birth and is unlikely to be influenced by maternal dietary deficiency. Hypocalcaemia is seen in babies born to diabetic mothers and in association with neonatal hypoglycaemia. It does not usually cause permanent brain damage, but is a common cause of neonatal tetany and/or convulsions.

20. A E

Polycystic ovarian syndrome (PCOS) is a disorder of multisystem involvement representing hypothalamic pituitary ovarian/adrenal interaction. Chronic stimulation by luteinising hormone (LH), compounded by hyper insulinaemia, combined with the overall increased amount of androgen secretory stromal and thecal tissue present in the ovary are major reasons for the excessive rate of ovarian androgen secretion in PCOS. Fasting insulin concentrations are raised in 33% of lean and 75% of obese women with PCOS. Insulin and possibly insulin-like growth factor 1 has a gonadotrophic action, promoting ovarian androgen synthesis and thus contributing to menstrual disturbances. Elevated levels of LH, leading to a hyperandrogenic environment within the follicle and premature ageing of the oocyte are suggested factors contributing to sub-fertility and poor pregnancy outcome in patients with PCOS.

21. C E

The commonest malignancy causing female deaths is breast cancer. There has not been a significant reduction in total mortality of women with cervical carcinoma in Great Britain. The incidence of the disease is increased in smokers. A Wertheim's hysterectomy is the usual treatment in a thin woman, but radiotherapy is used in the obese.

22. D E

Specific medical conditions.

In the recent handbook of the British Menopausal Society entitled *Management of the Menopause* published in 2002 the following links have been made between hormone replacement therapy and different conditions.

Condition	HRT
Fibroids	Can cause enlargement but evidence poor.
Endometriosis	Small increased risk of disease reactivation, but evidence poor.
Cervical cancer and dysplasia	Not contraindicated
Hypertension	Not contraindicated
Valvular heart disease	Not contraindicated
Hyperlipidaemia	Not contraindicated; route depends on lipid profile.
Diabetes mellitus	Increased risk of osteoporosis, not contraindicated.
Thyroid disease	Increased risk of osteoporosis; not contraindicated.
Migraine	Not contraindicated, transdermal route preferred.
Epilepsy	Not contraindicated, consider concomitant liver enzyme inducers and osteoporosis risk in phenytoin and carbamazepine users.
Parkinson's disease	May reduce risk of Parkinson's disease, not contraindicated.
Gall bladder disease	Increased risk
Liver disease	Transdermal route preferred; liaise with specialist.
Crohn's/coeliac disease	Increased risk osteoporosis; transdermal route preferred to enhance absorption.
Rheumatoid arthritis	Increased risk osteoporosis; no increase in flares.
Systemic lupus erythematosus	Increased risk osteoporosis; no increase in flares.
Asthma	Small increased risk; no worsening of pre-existing disease.
Otosclerosis	No evidence available to contraindicate.
Malignant melanoma	No association from epidemiological studies.
Post-transplant	Should be considered; increased risk osteoporosis.
Renal failure	Should be considered; increased risk early menopause.

Table reproduced from p.69 *Management of the Menopause*, The Handbook of the British Menopause Society, 3rd edition, 2002, with permission.

23. A B E

Down's syndrome involves an excess of chromosome 21 material usually due to trisomy, but in 4% of cases this does not amount to a separate chromosome. It most frequently arises due to non-separation of the chromosomes during meiosis. A female with Down's syndrome has a 1 in 2 chance of having a normal child. After the age of 40 the risk of an affected child is more than 1 in 100. Although the diagnosis of Down's syndrome should rest upon cytological culture from placenta or amniotic fluid and genetic studies, it may be associated with reduced serum α-fetoprotein.

24. B C D E

The placental barrier is completely effective against nearly all bacterial and protozoal invaders (*Toxoplasma* is an exception) and in general only viruses can cross it.

25. A B D

Prolonged physical contact is required in order for a scabies infestation to occur. The insect moves at a speed of approximately 25 mm per minute and, therefore, sexual contact needs to be reasonably prolonged. Symptoms can take up to 2–6 weeks after infestation to appear and the patient complains of itching, particularly worse at night when the body is warm. The diagnosis is made by finding the mite and this is achieved by scraping the top off the whole length of a burrow with a scalpel, putting the material on a slide with 10% potassium hydroxide solution and looking for the mite under the microscope.

26. A B D E

Gestational diabetes is a glucose intolerance that appears during pregnancy. Most cases can be treated by diet and there is no convincing evidence that insulin treatment of women with an abnormal glucose tolerance test will actually reduce the perinatal mortality. It does decrease the incidence of fetal macrosomia, but sadly there is no convincing evidence of a decrease in the incidence of operative delivery or birth trauma.

27. A B C

Luteinising hormone releasing hormone analogues saturate the receptors in the pituitary and therefore prevent recurrence of receptor function. This has been called the medical menopause, but this is a misnomer because the gonadotrophins will be low rather than high as is detected in the menopause. It therefore gives the endocrine picture of hypogonadotrophic hypogonadism, ie eventually low luteinising hormone, low follicle-stimulating hormone and a low oestradiol. The patient is likely to complain of menopausal symptoms, including hot flushes, night sweats, dry vagina as well as amenorrhoea. It is useful in the treatment of endometriosis, uterine fibroids and menorrhagia, but is not of long-term benefit because the side-effects of hypo-oestrogenism, ie osteoporosis, would otherwise occur. Long-term treatment with add-back therapy with tibolone has now been licensed. How long one can continue with this remains unclear.

28. B C

Oxygenated blood returns from the placenta via the umbilical vein; the umbilical arteries carry deoxygenated blood from fetus to placenta. The ductus venosus provides a direct route of flow for oxygenated blood from the umbilical vein to the inferior vena cava. The foramen ovale connects the atria and is an oblique passage through the interatrial septum, which closes soon after birth due to the greater left atrial pressure closing the septum primum against the septum secundum. The ductus arteriosus is a wide channel linking the left pulmonary artery with the aorta and joins the aorta distal to the origin of the three branches of the aortic arch.

29. C

The baby may appear well immediately after birth; signs usually develop within 1–2 hours. The chest X-ray appearances are suggestive, but not pathognomonic. Antibiotics are not indicated.

30. A D

Evidence-based medicine can sometimes bring surprise results. It is worth you reading the relevant sections in the BMJ Publishing Group, *Clinical Evidence* which is an international source of the best available evidence for effective health care.

In this book in the section hyperemesis the following is concluded:

Beneficial:	Antihistamines
Likely to be beneficial:	Cyanocobalamin (vitamin B12)
	Dietary ginger.
Unknown effectiveness:	Dietary intervention excluding ginger
	Acupressure
	Phenothiazines
	Pyridoxine (vitamin B6)
	Corticosteroids

31. C D

Genital warts are benign epidermal growths on the external perianal and perigenital region. They are caused by the human papillomavirus of which there are 70 types with types 6 and 11 usually being the causative factor in immunocompetent people.

Without treatment their natural life history is varied either staying the same, increasing in size, or spontaneously resolving. They rarely progress to cancer.

32. All True

In vulvodynia the majority of women presenting with vulval symptoms will be complaining of pruritus but a significant number will complain of vulval pain, burning and rawness.

The subsects of vulvodynia are:

- Vulvar dermatoses
- Cyclic vulvodynia
- Vestibular papillomatosis
- Vulvar vestibulitis
- Essential vulvodynia
- Idiopathic vulvodynia

33. A E

The important point about this question is the word 'screen'. Ultrasound scanning may be diagnostic for a non-genetic disease, such as spina bifida, but monitoring nuchal fold thickness may be beneficial as a screening test for Down's syndrome. Amniocentesis and chorionic villus sampling are both diagnostic tests rather than screening tests for genetic abnormalities. An X-ray would not be a useful screening test. α-fetoprotein, β-human chorionic gonadotrophin and oestriol are part of the triple test and may help screen for at-risk populations with Down's syndrome or other trisomies. α-fetoprotein and oestriol decrease in these instances, and β humanchorionic gonadotrophin increases. Recent research is directed towards a combination of ultrasound and biochemistry as a screening test.

34. A D

The exact incidence of pelvic inflammatory disease is unknown because the disease cannot be diagnosed reliably from clinical symptoms. Laparoscopy allows direct visualisation of the Fallopian tubes and is still the best single diagnostic test. It is not used routinely because it is invasive.

Pelvic inflammatory disease is the most common gynaecological reason for admission to hospital in the United States of America but most cases are asymptomatic. Most cases are a result of ascending infection from the cervix. The spread of the infection may be increased by vaginal douching and instrumentation of the cervix.

35. D E

This demonstrates the importance of reading the question. It states '... *in the third trimester...*'. In the first trimester vaginal scanning is an easier procedure than abdominal scanning, picks up pregnancies at an earlier gestation and does not require the uncomfortable full bladder. Biochemical tests for the assessment of fetal wellbeing have now fallen out of favour. This is especially due to delay in getting the result. On the basis of available studies there appears to be no good evidence that the measurement of human placental lactogen, oestriol, human chorionic gonadotrophin or α-fetoprotein in the third trimester are beneficial in the assessment of fetal wellbeing. A raised α-fetoprotein level at 16 weeks has a possible association with low birth weight, although the predictive value of this test is low. Less than 30% of the women with an abnormally high level of α-fetoprotein gave birth to a baby with low birth weight or low weight for gestational age. The usefulness of α-fetoprotein screening for conditions other than neural tube defects is poor. With the use of ultrasound scanning, the role of α-fetoprotein as a screening tool has been reduced. Biophysical tests are now playing a much more important role. These include fetal movement counting, non-stress cardiotocography and fetal bio-physical profiling. The role of fetal movement counting is controversial. It is known that there is a reduction or cessation of fetal movements that occurs in certain instances before fetal death, but this is by no means 100% predictive. The difficulty is that there are often huge vari-ations in the assessment of fetal kicking. There is also a question of whether, by monitoring the fetal movements, the mother is reassured; this can also have a negative effect in the mother putting some of the blame to herself if an abnormality is detected and not picked up. The non-stress cardiotocogram has been widely used in antenatal care. Doppler blood flow looking at the flow through the umbilical artery and other selective arteries of the baby is now being used as a routine method of assessing the fetus – it is more sensitive than cardiotoco-graphic monitoring.

36. C D E

Heart disease is potentially life threatening in pregnancy. Women with pulmonary vascular disease have a very high risk of dying in pregnancy.

Eisenmenger's syndrome has a mortality of 30%. Careful counselling must be given with the acceptance that there may be a cultural pressure to have a child. It is important to realise that women may minimise or even deny cardiac symptoms.

Endocarditis should always be on your differential with women with an obscure febrile illness.

Oxytocin must be used with caution with the risk of blood pressure changes and tachycardia. If oxytocin is required it should be given by a slow infusion and a maximum daily dose of 5 IU should not be exceeded.

37. All True

It was noted in the early 1970s that infants in the developing world who were fed formula had a much higher death rate than infants who were breast-fed. This was due to malnutrition and recurrent infectious diseases.

Breast-feeding is associated with decreased death rates due to acute respiratory infections and diarrhoea in infants aged 1–11 months in Bangladesh when compared to infants who were partially breast-fed. Breast-feeding was also found to be protective against enterotoxigenic *Escherichia coli* in the first year of life and associated with decreased incidence of *Giardia* infection.

Many anti-infective properties are found in breast milk including the following: Immunoglobulins IgA, IgM, IgG, lactoferrin, *Lactobacillis bifidus* growth factor, T and B cell lymphocytes, plasma cells and neutrophils.

Many studies show that exclusive breast-feeding for four months delayed the first episode of otitis media and decreased recurrent otitis media. In Britain studies showed breast-fed infants had fewer hospital admissions with bronchiolitis compared with nonbreast-fed infants.

38. All true

Oblique and transverse lies are associated with the fact that the fetus fails to adopt a longitudinal lie. This is associated with:

- The abdominal laxity of multiparity
- Congenital fetal abnormalities, especially those that cause polyhydramnios
- Uterine abnormalities, especially mild uterine abnormalities, such as subseptate uterus

- Shortening of the longitudinal axis of the uterus by fundal or low-lying placenta
- Conditions that prevent the engagement of the presenting part, including pelvic tumours and a small pelvic inlet.

39. A B D E

Growth restriction in later gestation and a low weight gain in infancy may be associated with an early menopause. It is interesting that the menopause occurs earlier in smokers and smoking causes a reduction in oestrogen. Remember the menopause is one day in a women's life, ie her last period. The climacteric is at the time when a women changes from being able to being unable to sexually reproduce.

40. All true

Ovarian hyperstimulation syndrome (OHSS) is a complication of induction of ovulation. It usually occurs after human chorionic gonadotrophin (hCG) has been given and also with luteal phase support with hCG. Women of a younger age, women with polycystic ovarian syndrome and those who have had a previous history of OHSS are at a higher risk. Early pregnancy which produces endogenous hCG is also a predisposing factor. Mild ovarian hyperstimulation presents with abdominal discomfort, swelling and pain and treatment is conservative. Moderate ovarian hyperstimulation often presents with nausea, vomiting and diarrhoea as well as weight gain. Severe hyperstimulation, which is rare, is more serious and pericardial and pleural effusions may develop. Close observation is very important and very careful fluid balance and electrolyte monitoring are essential. Fatalities are recognised, due not only to pulmonary embolism but also to renal failure.

41. A B D

Heartburn is a common condition in pregnancy. It is important to be aware that in late pregnancy it can be associated with pre-eclampsia and the HELLP syndrome. This syndrome stands for Haemolysis, Elevated Liver enzymes and Low Platelets. It is of the same pathophysiology as pre-eclampsia but may not have the initial rise in blood pressure. A useful screen blood test would include: liver function test, full blood count to include platelets, urea and electrolytes, urate.

42. D E

Biophysical profiling which measures fetal movement, tone, reactivity of the heart, breathing and amniotic fluid volume may be a better predictor of fetal compromise than cardiotocography alone. At present, it is a very time consuming and costly test and may not be appropriate as a screening test for fetal compromise. Although fetal biophysical profiling is a better predictor of low 5-minute Apgar scores than the non-stress test cardiotocogram, it does not, in its own right, reduce the perinatal mortality rate. Doppler blood flow assessment is now becoming routine clinical practice.

43. A C E
Condylomata acuminata are otherwise known as genital warts due to papillomavirus. Bartholinitis is usually caused by coliform organisms or staphylococci. Cervical intra-epithelial neoplasia (CIN) is thought to be caused by human papillomavirus, type 16. Lichen sclerosus is a type of vulval dystrophy of unknown aetiology. Acute vulval ulcers are most commonly due to infection by the herpes virus.

44. A B E
The most common symptom of cervical cancer is abnormal vaginal bleeding (such as postcoital bleeding, intermenstrual bleeding and postmenopausal bleeding. Studies demonstrate that human papillomavirus infection is the major risk factor for development of pre-invasive or invasive carcinoma of the cervix, which far outweighs other known risk factors such as increasing number of sexual partners, young age at first intercourse, low socioeconomic status, and positive smoking history. There were 2740 new cases of invasive cervical cancer in England and Wales in 1997 (9.3 cases per 100 000 women). The UK has the second highest recorded incidence in the European Union.

Deaths from cervical cancer have fallen by more than 40% from 7.0 deaths per 100 000 in 1979 to 4.1 per 100 000 in 1995. Cervical cancer is the 12th most common cause of cancer deaths in women in the UK.

45. B C E
Pregnancy induces a haemodilutionary effect on the blood and, therefore, the normal haemoglobin adaptations that occur with pregnancy may be inappropriately diagnosed as iron deficiency. Mean cell volume may be the most useful parameter for assessing iron deficiency as it falls quite rapidly in the presence of decreased iron. There is no good evidence that the addition of molybdenum, ascorbic acid, copper, or manganese improves the efficacy of iron. A megaloblastic anaemia in pregnancy is nearly always associated with folate deficiency with evidence of late-stage folate deficiency. Under

these circumstances rapid blood changes occur with folic acid supplementation.

46. A C E

The oral contraceptive pill has few side-effects. By increasing sex-hormone-binding-globulins it increases the bound testosterone and, therefore, decreases the testosterone activity. Danazol has an androgenic effect. Cyproterone acetate is most effective working at the level of the hair follicles as an anti-androgen and also decreasing gonadotrophin production. It needs to be given in an adequate dose and in a reversed sequential regime. There is no evidence that electrolysis increases the risk of further hair growth.

47. B C

Adequate contraception is important during the climacteric – that transitional phase during which ovarian function gradually ceases around the time of the final menstrual period (the menopause). Measurement of follicle-stimulating hormone (FSH) greater than 30 IU/l are usually suggestive of ovarian failure but one also has to be cautious about the diagnosis of resistant ovaries that can spontaneously ovulate. Reliable measurement of FSH can be difficult when a woman is using a combined oral contraceptive pill or taking hormone replacement therapy (HRT). HRT cannot be relied upon as a contraceptive as ovulation may still occur.

48. A

Vulval carcinoma is associated with pruritus vulvae. Pruritus vulvae is, however, a common problem associated with lichen sclerosis. Carcinoma of the vulva is increasing, but this is possibly associated with increasing life expectancy. Carcinoma of the vulva is usually unifocal, although it can be multifocal when 'KISS' lesions are noted. It is much more common in African patients and there is no association with parity. The treatment of choice is surgical.

49. A C D E

Abruption is a known complication of polyhydramnios due to the sudden decompression of the uterus at rupture of the membranes. It is essential when performing amniotomy to ensure that there is a slow release of the amniotic fluid. Intrauterine growth retardation results from poor uterine blood flow which causes placental insufficiency and oligohydramnios. Oesophageal atresia prevents effective fetal swallowing and therefore excessive amniotic fluid forms. The over-distended uterus is more irritable and therefore prone to preterm labour. The overstretched uterus does not retract and therefore post-partum haemorrhage is a complication in cases of polyhydramnios.

50. A B D

A progestogen is a steroid which causes a withdrawal bleed on an oestrogen-primed endometrium. If, when given to a postmenopausal woman, it induces a withdrawal bleed, endometrial hyperplasia should be suspected. Traditional therapy with cyclical oral progestogen is of limited efficiency in menorrhagia occurring during ovulatory cycles, unless the cycles are short. In this case, progestogens can help to delay the onset of bleeding. In prolonged cycles, progestogens may be useful, but side-effects are common and these include weight gain, nausea, bloating and headaches. Norethisterone has androgenic properties; medroxyprogesterone acetate and dydrogesterone are non-androgenic alternatives. Postmenopausal women are at risk of endometrial hyperplasia. If no uterus is present then unopposed oestrogen therapy is appropriate.

51. A E

Endometrial carcinoma tends to spread to lymphatics in the later stages or when there is extensive myometrial invasion. Radiotherapy is contraindicated in the presence of sepsis. Wertheim's hysterectomy entails the excision of uterus, tubes, often ovaries, upper third vagina, parametria and pelvic lymph nodes. The ovaries are excised in cases of carcinoma of the endometrium, as they are a site for malignant spread or oestrogen production and the disease usually occurs in the postmenopausal age group. Renal failure usually occurs in carcinoma of the cervix due to the tumour obstructing both ureters.

52. A B D E

Rubella, an RNA virus spread by droplet infection, is associated with a mild viral illness with macular papular rash and lymphadenopathy. Over 90% of women in the United Kingdom who attend antenatal clinics are immune to rubella. Toxoplasmosis is due to a protozoan, *Toxoplasma gondii*, and the oocysts are found in raw meat and cat faeces. It is a rare congenital infection occurring in approximately 1:100,000 births. Congenital infection occurs in 30% of infants whose mothers sero-convert during pregnancy and this can lead to stillbirth, neonatal death, or severe handicap. The treatment of choice is spiramycin. Varicella is a febrile illness in the mother, with a characteristic rash, a relation of the virus known as shingles. The congenital varicella syndrome, which is associated with skin scarring, is rare. *Listeria* is a Gram-positive bacillus associated with a non-specific febrile illness in the mother. It is specifically associated with soft cheeses and pre-packed food and occurs in approximately 1:700 pregnancies. It is associated with spontaneous abortion, stillbirth and neonatal death and can be treated with ampicillin.

53. A B D E

Dilatation and curettage (D&C) was the classical method of obtaining samples of the endometrium, having first been reported in 1843. In 1989–1990 it was one of the most common procedures performed, although it is increasingly being replaced by out-patient procedures as well as the use of the hysteroscope. A D&C does not sample all the endometrium and it has been shown that up to 5% of lesions are missed, including polyps, hyperplasia and even carcinoma. A D&C is not without risks and these include cervical tears, haemorrhage and even death following uterine perforation and damage to the bowel.

54. A B C D E

In uncomplicated vulvovaginal candidiasis topical antifungals will achieve clinical cure in 80% of cases. Oral azoles are contraindicated in pregnancy. Topical creams should also be used in conjunction with vaginal pessaries such as clotrimazole, econazole, or micronazole.

55. B C D

The rise in progesterone during pregnancy can cause a decrease in gut motility and thus constipation. Iron therapy can aggravate the problem.

56. B D

During pregnancy, fasting plasma glucose concentration is decreased, probably due to the haemodilution effect of the increased plasma volume. The glomerular filtration rate is increased in normal pregnancy; this may lead to the renal threshold being exceeded and to glycosuria without impaired glucose tolerance. Fasting plasma insulin concentration rises in late pregnancy to accompany the increased glucose requirements. Glucose tolerance alters during pregnancy; although plasma glucose levels should have returned to normal two hours after an oral glucose load, insulin concentration frequently remains elevated.

57. B C E

Androgen insensitivity syndrome is associated with chromosomal analysis of 46XY. Normally polycystic ovarian disease presents late, but it could be a possibility in this case. Primary ovarian failure would have higher luteinising and follicle-stimulating hormone levels. Imperforate hymen may be an option and the patient may also complain of cyclical pain as well as abdominal swelling.

58. C D

The organisms commonly responsible for meningitis in children and adults are relatively uncommon as a cause among the newborn.

59. B E

This booklet summarises the key findings and recommendations made in the Fifth Report of the Confidential Enquiries into Maternal Deaths in the United Kingdom 1997–99.

The key messages it contains are of relevance to all health professionals who plan or care for women during or after their pregnancy. These include GPs, midwives, obstetricians, staff in accident and emergency (A&E) departments, psychiatrists, anaesthetists and pathologists. The Confidential Enquiry into Maternal Deaths is the longest running example of national professional self-audit in the world. Women from the low socioeconomic class were about 20 times more likely to die than women in the highest social classes.

The maternal mortality rate for this triennium, derived from the CEMD data, is 11.4 deaths per 100 000 maternities. The direct maternal mortality rate is 5.0 deaths per 100 000 maternities. The indirect maternal mortality rate is 6.4 deaths per 100 000 maternities.

60. A B C E

The copper intrauterine device can cause an increase in menstrual blood loss, irregular bleeding and increased period pain.

MCQ Practice Exam 3

60 Questions: time allowed 2 hours. Indicate your answers clearly by putting a tick or cross against each answer option.

1. **Maternal mortality is significantly increased in the presence of**

   - [ ] **A** Marfan's syndrome
   - [ ] **B** valvular heart disease treated by curative surgery
   - [ ] **C** inoperable cyanotic congenital heart disease
   - [ ] **D** primary pulmonary hypertension
   - [ ] **E** congestive cardiomyopathy

2. **Causes of precocious puberty include**

   - [ ] **A** central neurological lesions
   - [ ] **B** polycystic ovarian syndrome
   - [ ] **C** chronic hyperthyroidism
   - [ ] **D** polycystic kidneys
   - [ ] **E** McCune–Albright syndrome

3. **Congenital varicella syndrome**

   - [ ] **A** is secondary to primary varicella zoster infections
   - [ ] **B** is associated with Down's syndrome
   - [ ] **C** is associated with skin scarring
   - [ ] **D** is associated with mental retardation
   - [ ] **E** occurs after 20 weeks' gestation

4. **Ovulation**

   - [ ] **A** is best assessed using basal body temperature
   - [ ] **B** is associated with a mid-luteal rise in progesterone
   - [ ] **C** can be demonstrated on an ultrasound scan
   - [ ] **D** can be detected by a rise in luteinising hormone
   - [ ] **E** is followed, after 12–16 days, by a withdrawal bleed if pregnancy does not occur

5. **Pre-eclampsia**

☐ **A** is most commonly found in women with their first pregnancy
☐ **B** is best treated with antihypertensive therapy and bed-rest
☐ **C** is negatively associated with smoking
☐ **D** has an increased incidence in diabetic pregnancies
☐ **E** the primary pathology is within the kidneys

6. **The following genetic conditions are sex-linked:**

☐ **A** The hairy pinna trait
☐ **B** Cleft palate
☐ **C** Hurler's syndrome (type I mucopolysaccharidosis)
☐ **D** Achondroplasia
☐ **E** Congenital ichthyosis

7. **Uterine fibroids**

☐ **A** need to be removed surgically in patients with secondary infertility
☐ **B** have an incidence of sarcomatous change of 1–2%
☐ **C** symptoms can be effectively treated medically
☐ **D** are more likely to occur after prolonged use of the oral contraceptive pill
☐ **E** are associated with heavy periods in more than 50% of cases

8. **The following statements regarding bone and the menopause are true:**

☐ **A** Osteoporosis is a systematic skeletal disease characterised by microarchitectural deterioration of bone tissue with resultant decreased fragility
☐ **B** Approximately 15% of women aged above 50 have osteoporosis
☐ **C** Osteopenia is defined as bone mineral density less than −1.0 SD below the young adult mean to less than −2.5 SD
☐ **D** Osteoporosis is defined as a bone mineral density of ≥ -2.5 SD below the young adult mean
☐ **E** The T score is a value that has been defined based on a mean axial bone mineral density relative to the patient's chronological age

9. **The following are recognised causes of recurrent spontaneous abortion:**

   ☐ **A** Polycystic ovarian syndrome
   ☐ **B** Maternal diabetes
   ☐ **C** Maternal brucella infection
   ☐ **D** Chromosomal abnormalities of the fetus
   ☐ **E** Intercourse

10. **The following drugs cross the placental barrier:**

   ☐ **A** Heparin
   ☐ **B** Tetracycline
   ☐ **C** Sulphadimidine
   ☐ **D** Diazepam
   ☐ **E** Salicylate

11. **A cervical eversion**

   ☐ **A** is often found in postmenopausal women
   ☐ **B** should always be investigated by cervical smear
   ☐ **C** can cause chronic vaginal discharge
   ☐ **D** if asymptomatic, should still be treated
   ☐ **E** can be treated with coagulation of the cervix

12. **The following statements about the management of genital herpes in pregnancy are true:**

   ☐ **A** Concern is raised because of neonatal herpes
   ☐ **B** If a woman presents with the first attack of genital herpes, referral to a genitourinary physician should be made.
   ☐ **C** Treatment with acyclovir should be considered for women with first attack
   ☐ **D** Caesarean section is the mode of choice for all women who present with first attack of genital herpes in the first trimester
   ☐ **E** For women presenting with recurrent genital herpes lesion, the risk to the baby is small

13. **The vaginal contraceptive diaphragm**

   ☐ **A** is graded in 15 mm sizes
   ☐ **B** should be removed within two hours of intercourse
   ☐ **C** is recommended in case of prolapse
   ☐ **D** should be checked if the patient's weight changes by more than 7 lb
   ☐ **E** should be replaced annually

14. The following statements about eclampsia are true:

- [ ] **A** Incidence in UK is 4.9/10 000 maternities
- [ ] **B** 44% of eclampsias occur postnatally
- [ ] **C** 38% of eclampsias occur antepartum
- [ ] **D** Maternal fatality rate is 1.8%
- [ ] **E** 35% of women will have one major complication

15. The baby of a diabetic mother runs

- [ ] **A** an increased risk of congenital heart disease compared to a baby from a non-diabetic mother
- [ ] **B** a five-fold increase in risk of respiratory distress syndrome
- [ ] **C** a 10% risk of developing diabetes
- [ ] **D** a greatly increased risk of mental retardation
- [ ] **E** a risk of hypomagnesaemia in the neonatal period

16. The following are evidence-based treatment options for endometriosis causing pain:

- [ ] **A** Non-steroidal drugs
- [ ] **B** Combined oral contraceptive
- [ ] **C** Gonadotrophin-releasing hormone agonist
- [ ] **D** Laparoscopic ablation
- [ ] **E** Continuous progestogens

17. The fetal head

- [ ] **A** may be at the ischial spines but not engaged
- [ ] **B** can be delivered vaginally in a mento-posterior position
- [ ] **C** will display Spalding's sign within 24 hours of intrauterine death
- [ ] **D** may undergo asynclitism in negotiating the pelvic outlet
- [ ] **E** is likely to be a vertex presentation when deflexed

18. Human chorionic gonadotrophin

- [ ] **A** is produced by the trophoblast
- [ ] **B** is produced by the fetal liver
- [ ] **C** may be immunosuppressive
- [ ] **D** the serum level peaks in the second trimester of pregnancy
- [ ] **E** is produced by some non-trophoblastic tumours

19. In the menstrual cycle

- ☐ **A** ovulation follows the luteinising hormone surge by 48 hours
- ☐ **B** oestradiol stimulates endometrial cell proliferation in the proliferative phase
- ☐ **C** progesterone, in the secretory phase, produces vacuolation of the cell with the nuclei displaced towards the gland lumen
- ☐ **D** the bleed is caused by failure of implantation and a cessation of oestrogen production
- ☐ **E** early production of trophoblastic human chorionic gonadotrophin maintains the corpus luteum and thus prevents the withdrawal bleed

20. Endometrial carcinoma

- ☐ **A** frequently occurs in women aged 30–34
- ☐ **B** is associated with unopposed progestogens
- ☐ **C** is treated by radiotherapy
- ☐ **D** can be diagnosed by ultrasound scanning
- ☐ **E** has a poor prognosis

21. The following are correct for Apgar scores:

- ☐ **A** Heart rate: >100 bpm = 2
- ☐ **B** Colour: blue and pale = 0
- ☐ **C** Muscle tone: some limb flexion = 1
- ☐ **D** Respiratory effort: slow and irregular = 1
- ☐ **E** Eye movement: irregular = 0

22. The following statements about an ectopic pregnancy are true:

- ☐ **A** It is very rarely associated with *in vitro* fertilisation
- ☐ **B** The diagnosis can be excluded by ultrasound scanning
- ☐ **C** Surgery is the only treatment
- ☐ **D** Is associated with maternal death
- ☐ **E** It can be excluded if a gestational sac is seen within the uterus

23. A raised serum α-fetoprotein is likely in the following conditions:

- ☐ **A** Spina bifida occulta
- ☐ **B** Down's syndrome
- ☐ **C** Threatened abortion
- ☐ **D** Exomphalos
- ☐ **E** Multiple pregnancy

24. Bacterial vaginosis

- [ ] **A** is less common than candida
- [ ] **B** is caused by the lactobacilli
- [ ] **C** creates a pH of the vagina greater than 4.5
- [ ] **D** is associated with a fishy odour
- [ ] **E** may be associated with preterm labour

25. The typical female bony pelvis

- [ ] **A** has a transverse diameter at the inlet greater than the antero-posterior diameter
- [ ] **B** has an obstetric conjugate of 11–12 cm
- [ ] **C** is funnel-shaped
- [ ] **D** has an obtuse greater sciatic notch
- [ ] **E** has a subpubic angle greater than 90°

26. Fetal pulmonary maturity

- [ ] **A** is delayed in diabetic pregnancies
- [ ] **B** normally occurs before the 36th week of gestation
- [ ] **C** is influenced by corticosteroid levels
- [ ] **D** is controlled by α-fetoprotein
- [ ] **E** is always delayed in cases of growth retardation

27. The following tumours arise in the ovary:

- [ ] **A** Nephroblastoma
- [ ] **B** Cystadenoma
- [ ] **C** Granulosa cell tumour
- [ ] **D** Neuroblastoma
- [ ] **E** Teratoma

28. Amniocentesis in the second trimester

- [ ] **A** is associated with an overall pregnancy loss more than 3% that of matched controls
- [ ] **B** carries a greater risk of fetal wastage when the placenta is implanted anteriorly as opposed to posteriorly
- [ ] **C** is indicated in a woman whose female cousin has previously delivered a child with a neural tube defect
- [ ] **D** carries a diagnostic error rate of around 10% in chromosomal analysis
- [ ] **E** is associated with a 2% risk of failure of the cells to culture

29. *Chlamydia trachomatis*

- [ ] **A** has an intracellular existence
- [ ] **B** causes psittacosis
- [ ] **C** is associated with Fitzhugh–Curtis syndrome
- [ ] **D** is best treated by penicillin derivatives
- [ ] **E** can only be detected by the measurement of a heat-stable antigen

30. Regarding postpartum haemorrhage (PPH):

- [ ] **A** The most frequent cause of PPH is uterine atony
- [ ] **B** Risk factors include previous PPH
- [ ] **C** Primary PPH occurs within 72 hours after delivery
- [ ] **D** Secondary PPH occurs in approximately 10% of all deliveries
- [ ] **E** Intramuscular or intramyometrial prostaglandin (Hemabate; 0.25 mg) can be used for uterine atony

31. Nausea and vomiting

- [ ] **A** are among the most troublesome symptoms of early pregnancy
- [ ] **B** in early pregnancy are usually due to a rise in oestrogen levels
- [ ] **C** can be treated with antihistamines which are considered to be safe in pregnancy
- [ ] **D** in late pregnancy can be associated with pre-eclampsia
- [ ] **E** can be the presenting feature of a hydatidiform mole

32. Premature ovarian failure may be due to:

- [ ] **A** Chromosome abnormalities
- [ ] **B** Autoimmune disease
- [ ] **C** Metabolic disease
- [ ] **D** Chemotherapy
- [ ] **E** Hysterectomy and conservation of ovaries

33. In the days following ovulation

- [ ] **A** the basal body temperature falls
- [ ] **B** the endometrium undergoes secretory changes
- [ ] **C** the plasma progesterone concentration falls
- [ ] **D** cervical mucus becomes scanty and more viscous
- [ ] **E** plasma luteinising hormone level falls

34. Concerning antepartum haemorrhage

☐ **A** it may be due to a cervical eversion
☐ **B** it may be treated with rest at home if the cervix is closed
☐ **C** rhesus-negative patients should be given anti-D immunoglobulin
☐ **D** it is associated with an increased incidence of postpartum haemorrhage
☐ **E** if due to placental abruption, blood loss is a good indicator of severity

35. The following should be discussed with a female patient before one agrees to carry out a sterilisation:

☐ **A** that there is a failure rate of approximately 10%
☐ **B** that she is aware that reversal is possible
☐ **C** that it is routinely performed by laparoscopic electrodiathermy of the tubes
☐ **D** that it will make her periods heavier
☐ **E** that her partner has considered a vasectomy

36. Increasing maternal age is associated with

☐ **A** an increased risk of Down's syndrome
☐ **B** a decreased risk of miscarriage
☐ **C** a decreased risk of monozygotic twins
☐ **D** an increased risk of hydatidiform moles
☐ **E** a decreased risk of postpartum haemorrhage

37. Genital herpes

☐ **A** is usually caused by the same organism as lip herpes
☐ **B** is often recurrent
☐ **C** is usually transmitted sexually
☐ **D** if uncomplicated will heal without treatment in about 10 days
☐ **E** should be treated with penicillin if secondary infection develops

38. **The following statements about perimenopausal contraception are true:**

  ☐ **A** Female sterilisation is the most commonly used method of contraception in the age group 40–49 years.
  ☐ **B** Women should stop the combined oral contraceptive pill (COCP) at the age of 45.
  ☐ **C** Progestogen-only pill (POP) should only be used in women for whom the combined oral contraceptive pill is contraindicated
  ☐ **D** A copper-containing intrauterine device inserted after the age of 40 can be left until contraception is no longer required
  ☐ **E** Emergency combined hormonal contraception can be used in this group

39. **The following definitions are correct:**

  ☐ **A** Secondary amenorrhoea: the absence of menses for six months in a previously menstruating woman
  ☐ **B** Dysfunctional uterine bleeding: excessive or prolonged regular menstrual bleeding in the absence of overt uterine, endocrine, or haematological disorder
  ☐ **C** Climacteric: the last menstrual period
  ☐ **D** Puberty: the first menstrual period
  ☐ **E** Dysmenorrhoea: painful vaginal bleeding

40. **In 'Why Mothers Die 1997–1999':**

  ☐ **A** Thrombosis and thromboembolism remain the major indirect causes of maternal death
  ☐ **B** Thrombosis and thromboembolism account for 33% of all direct maternal deaths
  ☐ **C** Hypertensive disease of pregnancy remains the third leading cause of direct deaths
  ☐ **D** Sepsis, including deaths in early pregnancy following miscarriage and ectopic pregnancy, is the third leading cause of direct death
  ☐ **E** Deaths in early pregnancy are the second leading cause of direct deaths

41. **The following statements about low-dose aspirin and pregnancy are true:**

   □ **A** The usual dose is 75 mg/day
   □ **B** It is associated with an increased risk of accidental haemorrhage
   □ **C** It is useful in preventing the deterioration of pre-eclampsia
   □ **D** It may be useful in the prevention of recurrent miscarriage
   □ **E** It may be useful in thromboprophylaxis

42. *Gardnerella vaginalis*

   □ **A** is a Gram-negative bacillus
   □ **B** is associated with clue cells which are bacteria attached to vaginal epithelial cells
   □ **C** is associated with a vaginal pH >5
   □ **D** can be transported on Stuart's medium
   □ **E** generates a strawberry odour

43. **Important guidelines for the management of recurrent vulvovaginal candidiasis include:**

   □ **A** Symptoms of thrush are typically worse before and better after menstruation
   □ **B** Advice re. avoidance of tightly fitting synthetic garments should be given
   □ **C** Treatment regimes that work well in cases of uncomplicated thrush may be ineffective in recurrent thrush
   □ **D** Clotrimazole 500 mg vaginally weekly is a useful maintenance therapy
   □ **E** Maintenance therapy should be given for no longer than one month

44. **Ultrasound in pregnancy**

   □ **A** detected anencephaly for the first time in 1971
   □ **B** has reduced perinatal deaths not due to congenital abnormality
   □ **C** can be used to screen for Down's syndrome
   □ **D** is a safe procedure
   □ **E** can be done in early pregnancy by use of a vaginal probe

45. Puerperal psychosis

- ☐ **A** usually begins after the second week of the puerperium
- ☐ **B** often takes the form of schizophrenia
- ☐ **C** recurs in subsequent pregnancies as a rule
- ☐ **D** usually develops insidiously
- ☐ **E** usually has a good prognosis

46. Fetal size and growth

- ☐ **A** is accurately measured by abdominal palpation
- ☐ **B** is best assessed by an ultrasound scan
- ☐ **C** is closely related to maternal weight gain
- ☐ **D** is usefully screened using fundal height measurement
- ☐ **E** will vary between different racial groups

47. *Why Mothers Die 1997–1999*: in comparison with the report from 1994–96, the overall findings for 1997–99 show:

- ☐ **A** Increased deaths from pulmonary embolism
- ☐ **B** Significant decrease in deaths from sepsis following Caesarean section
- ☐ **C** Number of direct deaths is greater than number of indirect maternal deaths
- ☐ **D** Deaths from suicide are the leading cause of maternal deaths
- ☐ **E** The total number of deaths remarkably similar to that reported in 1994–96

48. Preterm rupture of membranes (PROM):

- ☐ **A** occurs in one out of ten pregnancies after 37 weeks
- ☐ **B** preterm premature rupture of the membranes (PPROM) occurs before 37 weeks and after the onset of labour
- ☐ **C** can lead to premature delivery
- ☐ **D** presents with the main complaint being of pelvic pressure
- ☐ **E** can be managed expectantly

49. Analgesia in labour

- ☐ **A** Epidural analgesia is the most effective method
- ☐ **B** It is likely that epidural analgesia lengthens labour and results in increased rates of operative vaginal delivery
- ☐ **C** Nitrous oxide is commonly the inhalation analgesia used
- ☐ **D** Transcutaneous nerve stimulation (TENS) can be used in labour
- ☐ **E** Pethidine is a central nervous system depressant

50. Lactation and infant feeding:

- ☐ **A** Breast-feeding protects again gastrointestinal infection in the infant
- ☐ **B** Combined oestrogen–progestogen oral contraceptives should not be avoided in breast-feeding mothers
- ☐ **C** Oestrogen can be used to suppress lactation
- ☐ **D** Carbergoline is more effective than bromocriptine for the suppression of lactation and may be used as a single dose
- ☐ **E** Antibiotics and/or cabbage leaves are very effective for breast engorgement

51. The principles of antenatal care:

- ☐ **A** Dietary advice should focus on a well-balanced and varied diet, such as raw meat and soft cheeses
- ☐ **B** Vigorous exercise should be limited to one hour daily
- ☐ **C** Pelvic floor exercises should be included in all antenatal exercise programmes
- ☐ **D** A minimum of four antenatal visits is recommended for a woman with a normal pregnancy
- ☐ **E** The early antenatal care is important in the prevention and treatment of anaemia

52. Pruritus vulvae

- ☐ **A** is the same as vulvodynia
- ☐ **B** can be caused by lichen sclerosis
- ☐ **C** is suffered by 1% of women world-wide
- ☐ **D** is contributed to by glycosuria and diabetes
- ☐ **E** occurs as a result of purulent and mucopurulent vaginal discharge in 20% of cases

53. Vulvodynia:

- ☐ **A** is known as vulvar vestibulitis syndrome
- ☐ **B** is defined as acute vulval pain
- ☐ **C** often occurs in a vagina that shows no abnormalities
- ☐ **D** occurs only on provocation, such as with attempted vaginal penetration for sexual intercourse
- ☐ **E** has a prevalence as high as 15%

54. Induction of labour:

- [ ] **A** Induction of labour can be conducted on antenatal wards
- [ ] **B** Cardiotocogram should be performed prior to induction of labour
- [ ] **C** Prolonged use of maternal facial oxygen therapy should be used whenever needed
- [ ] **D** Continuous cardiotocography should not be used with induction of labour with oxytocin
- [ ] **E** Women with uncomplicated pregnancies should be offered induction of labour prior to 41 weeks

55. Signs and symptoms of pregnancy:

- [ ] **A** Hegar's sign, a softening of the lower third of the vagina, occurs around six weeks
- [ ] **B** Physical signs during the first trimester are reliable predictors of pregnancy
- [ ] **C** Average duration of pregnancy is 266 days from ovulation date
- [ ] **D** Enlargement of the uterus begins eight weeks after implantation
- [ ] **E** Half of pregnant women will experience nausea and vomiting in the first trimester

56. Fertilisation and implantation:

- [ ] **A** Fertilisation occurs six hours after ovulation
- [ ] **B** Implantation usually occurs within about 48 hours of ovulation
- [ ] **C** Fertilisation usually occurs in the ampulla
- [ ] **D** The most common site of abnormal implantation is in the uterine tube
- [ ] **E** Spermatogenesis occurs in the seminiferous tubules of testes and begins at the time of birth

57. β-human chorionic gonadotrophin (β-hCG):

- [ ] **A** Trophoblastic cells produce hCG
- [ ] **B** hCG levels double every 1.3–2 days
- [ ] **C** Modern urine pregnancy tests can detect hCG concentrations as low as 5 mIU/ml
- [ ] **D** Urine pregnancy tests can be positive three days after implantation
- [ ] **E** Radioimmunoassay techniques for measuring serum β-hCG can detect levels as low as 2 mIU/ml

58. Risk factors for ectopic pregnancy include:

- [ ] **A** previous history of pelvic inflammatory disease
- [ ] **B** previous tubal surgery
- [ ] **C** previous ectopic pregnancy
- [ ] **D** intrauterine contraceptive device (coil) *in situ*
- [ ] **E** *in vitro* fertilisation (IVF) treatment or assisted fertilisation

59. Serum human chorionic gonadotrophin (hCG):

- [ ] **A** can be positive within 7–10 days of conception
- [ ] **B** doubles approximately every 48 hours in 85% of normal intrauterine pregnancies of 4–6 weeks
- [ ] **C** rises <66% in 48 hours in more than 80% of ectopic pregnancies
- [ ] **D** at levels of 500 IU/L should normally indicate a visible intrauterine sac
- [ ] **E** may also be increased with certain types of ovarian tumors and testicular tumors

60. Risk factors for cord prolapse include:

- [ ] **A** multiple pregnancy
- [ ] **B** breech presentation
- [ ] **C** transverse and oblique lie
- [ ] **D** polyhydramnios
- [ ] **E** pre-term labour

MCQ Practice Exam 3: Answers and Teaching Notes

1. **A C D E**
   Patients who have undergone curative cardiac surgery are at no increased risk. It is important to get the cardiologist involved in the antenatal care. The remaining conditions are all associated with increased maternal mortality and are grounds for the doctor to consider counselling the patient to avoid pregnancy altogether.

2. **A C E**
   Precocious puberty is much more common in girls than in boys and may commence at any age from infancy onwards. Accelerated linear growth is usually its first manifestation. Precocious puberty can be broken up into central precocious puberty, ie the hypothalamic pituitary axis is activated, and precocious pseudo-puberty when the normal endocrine axis is inactive. True central precocious puberty can be constitutional without any evidence of disorder. This occurs close to the normal time of puberty and is often familial. Idiopathic true precocious puberty is a diagnosis of exclusion and is much more common in girls than in boys. Several neurological disorders can induce early activation of the hypothalamic reproductive axis. Tumours, such as hypothalamic hamartoma and astrocytomas, may also cause this. Previous central nervous insults, such as hydrocephalus, cranial irradiation, infections or skull trauma, may also induce precocious puberty. All cause early release from central inhibition of the endocrine axis and must be considered in the differential diagnosis. Chronic hyperthyroidism is thought to induce central precocious puberty by thyroid stimulating hormone/luteinising hormone overlap. Precocious pseudo-puberty is most often caused by oestrogen coming from another source. McCune–Albright syndrome refers to polyostotic fibrous dysplasia characterised by multiple cystic lesions of the skull and long bones, a propensity to fracture, café-au-lait skin patches and a predisposition to other endocrine hypersecretion disorders. Some follicular cysts secrete enough oestrogen to induce precocious puberty, but this is not associated with the polycystic ovarian syndrome. Granulosa tumours of the ovary may do the same. Some adrenal tumours are also

said to feminise rather than virilise, but these are very rare. Exogenous oestradiol from medications, such as contraceptive pills, or eating meat from oestrogen-treated animals, should not be forgotten as an occasional source of exposure.

3. **A C D**

Congenital varicella zoster is secondary to primary varicella zoster infection occurring before 20 weeks' gestation.

The syndrome includes one or more of the following:

a. Skin scarring in a dermatomal distribution
b. Eye defects (microphthalmia, chorioretinitis and cataracts)
c. Hypoplasia of the limbs
d. Neurological abnormalities,

microcephaly, cortical atrophy, mental retardation and dysfunction of bowel and bladder sphincters.

The risk is about 2% and does not occur if the primary maternal infection occurs after 20 weeks' gestation.

4. **B C D E**

The only definite ways to confirm ovulation are by a pregnancy or by picking the oocyte up from the pouch of Douglas. Basal body temperature has a limited role. Other methods of detecting ovarian activity include:

- Changes in cervical mucus with pre-ovulatory cervical mucus clear, acellular and having low viscosity. On the day of ovulation Spinnbarkeit can occur with threads of cervical mucus reaching up to 15–20 cm without breaking.
- Endometrial biopsy demonstrating secretory changes.
- Laparoscopy which can show the corpus luteum.
- Ultrasound scan with sequential ultrasound scanning demonstrating growth of the dominant follicle, rupture and then development of the corpus luteum.
- A rise in the luteinising hormone mid-cycle and a mid-luteal phase progesterone peak are associated with ovulation.

5. **A C D**

Pre-eclampsia is a multi-system disorder having the potential to affect all the systems of the body, including the placenta and the fetus. The prime pathology is an abnormal relationship between the maternal system and the trophoblastic system. It has a greater incidence in diabetic pregnancies, multiple pregnancies and hydatidiform moles. It is interesting that patients who smoke have a lower incidence of pre-eclampsia. It is generally a disease of women in their first pregnancy, but a miscarriage from the same relationship may, in some way, be protective.

6. **A E**
    The term 'sex-linkage' is virtually synonymous with X-linkage; the Y chromosome appears to have few loci apart from those determining the male sex. The only documented Y-linked state is that of the 'hairy pinna'. Congenital ichthyosis is an X-linked disorder associated with a steroid sulphatase deficiency (and hence may be associated with very low oestriol levels in pregnancy). Hurler's syndrome is determined by an autosomal recessive gene and achondroplasia by an autosomal dominant gene. Cleft palate, whether or not associated with cleft lip, seems to have a multifactorial inheritance pattern.

7. **C**
    Uterine fibroids are benign growths of the myometrium. There are many different forms of treatment and presentation, but presentation usually includes heavy periods as well as pain, dyspareunia, irregular bleeding and infertility. Medical treatment includes the use of the luteinising hormone-releasing hormone analogue which does reduce the size of the fibroid, but the size may increase after discontinuation. Fibroids are dependent on oestrogen and it may be that oestrogen abnormality causes the heavy periods rather than the original theory of an increased surface area. Surgical treatment is possible and this may be done with a resectoscope as well as by an open myomectomy. Sarcomatous change is rare. Embolisation of the artery that feeds the fibroid has now been demonstrated to be effective. It does have complications including a risk of hysterectomy. At present it is not suitable for women wanting to maintain their fertility.

8. **B C D E**
    Osteoporosis leads to INCREASED fragility – read the question! The T score is the bone mineral density in a healthy young adult female population.

9. **A B C D**
    Polycystic ovarian syndrome is associated with recurrent spontaneous abortion, probably due to the raised basal luteinising hormone. The most common cause of spontaneous abortion is chromosomal abnormalities. These may be recurrent, especially in the older woman and those with a balanced translocation.

10. B C D E

The injectable anticoagulant, heparin, is the anticoagulant of choice in pregnancy because it is a large molecule and does not cross the placenta as most oral anticoagulants do. Tetracycline is contraindicated in pregnancy because it does cross the placenta. Adverse effects include deposition in and staining of deciduous teeth and bones, tooth malformations and decrease in linear bone growth. Sulphadimidine rapidly crosses from mother to fetus. If given immediately before delivery there is a theoretical risk of competition between sulphonamides and bilirubin for binding sites on neonatal albumin. Diazepam readily crosses the placenta, whichever route of administration is used, and can cause behavioural problems for many hours after birth if given in late pregnancy or labour. Salicylates cross the placenta and can cause neonatal platelet dysfunction, decreased neonatal factor XII, neonatal haemorrhage and respiratory distress syndrome.

11. C E

A cervical eversion is also called a cervical ectropion. This is an eversion of the squamocolumnar junction which is present in the lower cervical canal. This gives a florid appearance to the cervix and commonly occurs during adolescence, pregnancy, and whilst taking the combined oral contraceptive pill (ie in states of increased oestrogenisation). The term erosion is a misnomer because this does imply an eroded area which would be present in carcinoma. A cervical smear may be indicated before any treatment, but if one is suspicious of cancer of the cervix, a cervical biopsy is the management. Twenty per cent of cervical carcinomas have negative smears and a cervical smear is, therefore, a screening test for premalignant and not for malignant disease. Cervical erosions may be asymptomatic, but can cause a variety of symptoms, including chronic vaginal discharge, intermenstrual bleeding and postcoital bleeding. Treatment should only be carried out if the patient is symptomatic.

12. A B C E

Neonatal herpes is a secure systemic viral infection with a high morbidity which is most commonly acquired at or near the time of delivery (RCOG Clinical Green Top Guideline). There is no clinical or laboratory evidence of fetal toxicity with acyclovir and this is known to help reduce the duration and severity of symptoms as well as decrease the duration of viral shedding. Caesarean section is recommended for all women presenting with the first episode of genital herpes at the time of delivery.

13. D E

The diaphragm is graded in 5 mm sizes and it should be left in position for at least six hours after intercourse. In cases of prolapse a good diaphragm fitting is not possible.

14. All True

The primary cause of eclampsia is unknown but cerebral vasospasm, ischaemia and oedema are the main effects. Neurological complications include:

- Coma
- Focal motor deficits
- Cortical blindness
- Cerebrovascular haemorrhage

Eclampsia is part of a multisystem disorder and associated complications include:

- HELLP (Haemolysis, elevated liver enzymes and low platelets) 3%
- Disseminated intravascular coagulation 3%
- Renal failure 4%
- Adult respiratory distress syndrome 3%

15. A B E

The risk of the child developing diabetes is thought to be 1–5%. Mental retardation is uncommon. The blood levels of both calcium and magnesium may fall significantly during the first three days of life if the mother is being treated with insulin; this is thought to be due to delayed development of the baby's parathyroid function.

16. All True

In a recent publication by the RCOG (Investigation and Management of Endometriosis Guideline 24 July 2000) they indicated that if a woman is not trying to conceive and there is no evidence of a pelvic mass on examination, there may be a role for a therapeutic trial of a combined oral contraceptive (monthly or tricycling) or a progestogen to treat pain symptoms suggestive of endometriosis without performing a diagnostic laparoscopy first. The choice between the combined oral contraceptive pill, progestogens, danazol and gonadotrophin-releasing hormone (GnRH) agonists depends principally on their side-effects profiles because they relieve pain associated with endometriosis equally well. GnRH agonist therapy given for three months may be as effective as treatment given for six months in relieving endometriosis-associated pain. Using GnRH agonists for greater than six months increases the risks of osteoporosis but add-back therapy can be given.

17. A

The head may be at the ischial spines when there is a large caput. It is important to perform abdominal palpation at the same time as vaginal examination. A mento-posterior face presentation will not be able to traverse the birth canal because flexion will not occur. Conversely, in a mento-anterior position flexion may result in a subsequent vaginal delivery. Spalding's sign, overlapping of the skull bones due to fetal death in utero, tends to appear by about 3–7 days. Asynclitism is the phenomenon by which the head negotiates the pelvic inlet by a rocking method where one parietal bone leads the other. When the head is deflexed, it is not likely to be a vertex, but a malpresentation, eg face or brow.

18. A C E

Human chorionic gonadotrophin (hCG) is produced by the placental trophoblast and some other tissues but not by the fetal liver. The level in maternal serum rises rapidly in early pregnancy reaching a peak between eight and ten weeks of pregnancy. There is then a rapid reduction to 18 weeks, after which levels remain more or less constant until delivery. hCG almost certainly rescues the corpus luteum from dissolution and promotes placental steroidogenesis. It is also important in the induction of fetal testosterone secretion by Leydig cells in the male fetus. It is suggested that hCG mediates the immuno-logical privilege afforded to the fetus. A variety of gonadal and non-gonadal tumours have been reported to produce hCG; these include tumours of the lung, stomach, liver, breast, kidney, pancreas, ovary and testis, carcinoid tumours and lymphomas.

19. B C E

Ovulation occurs within 24 hours of the luteinising hormone surge. Oestradiol causes endometrial cell division and this is why it is called proliferation. The proliferative phase can lead to a thickness of the endometrium, up to 6–8 mm in depth. Progesterone causes a with-drawal bleed on an oestrogen-primed endometrium. It is, therefore, not the cessation of oestrogen production, but cessation of proges-terone production. Trophoblastic human chorionic gonadotrophin maintains the life of the corpus luteum which otherwise has a limited lifespan of 12–16 days, thus preventing the withdrawal bleed.

20. None Correct

The incidence of endometrial carcinoma in women aged between 30 and 34 is 0.66 per 100 000 women. Endometrial carcinoma is asso-ciated with unopposed oestrogens. The incidence is in the order of

6% after five years' use of unopposed oestrogens, rising to 22% after 10 years. As it is usually detected early, with postmenopausal bleeding or irregular bleeding, the prognosis is good and the treatment is generally surgery followed by radiotherapy in some cases. Endometrial carcinoma is not usually diagnosed by ultrasound scanning; a thick endometrium in a woman who is postmenopausal is suggestive of it, but not diagnostic.

21. A B C D

Apgar scores	0	1	2
Heart rate	absent	<100 bpm	>100 bpm
Respiratory effort	absent	weak, irregular	strong cry
Muscle tone	limp	some limb flexion	active motion
Reflex irritability response on suctioning the pharynx	no	grimace	cough or cry
Colour	pale/overall cyanosis	peripherally blue, centrally pink	pink all over

22. D

The incidence of ectopic pregnancy is increased to about 3% in conceptions following in vitro fertilisation or gamete intrafallopian transfer. Suspicions should be raised in anybody who misses a period and easy access to β-human chorionic gonadotrophin pregnancy testing units is essential. Different forms of surgical treatment available include laparoscopic removal, salpingostomy, but may include a salpingectomy. Medical treatment has been, and still is, under investigation, including injection of methotrexate into the sac.

23. C D E

Open neural tissue in the fetus will result in the passage of fetal proteins into the maternal circulation. Spina bifida occulta is a closed lesion, so this will not cause a rise in the α-fetoprotein level. Down's syndrome may be associated with low serum levels of α-fetoprotein. Threatened abortion may result in fetal–maternal transfusion, hence the presence of fetal blood will raise maternal serum α-fetoprotein. Multiple pregnancy will cause a rise in α-fetoprotein, the exact mechanism of this is unknown but presumably reflects the increased amount of fetal tissue.

24. C D E

Bacterial vaginosis is the most common infective cause of vaginitis, being twice as common as candida. It is a microbial disease due to decrease in the *Lactobacillus* species and an increase in anaerobic bacteria. There is a high incidence in lesbians.

Diagnosis requires three of the following four features:

- Presence of clue cells
- Homogeneous discharge adherent to vagina walls.
- pH in vagina greater than 4.5
- Fishy smell especially if potassium hydroxide added

Symptoms include:

- Asymptomatic in 50% of cases
- Excessive white-grey discharge
- Odour is notable post-sexual intercourse

25. A B D E

The typical female pelvis in the Caucasian has a brim which is slightly wider in its transverse than its anteroposterior diameter (gynaecoid), the true obstetric conjugate being 11–12 cm and the transverse 13 cm. The cavity has the contours of a curved cylinder rather than a funnel, the side walls being approximately parallel. The greater sciatic notch is usually greater than 90° and the subpubic angle should also approximate to a right angle.

26. A B C

Fetal lung alveoli are lined by a group of phospholipids known collectively as surfactant, which prevent collapse of the alveoli during respiration by reducing surface tension. The predominant phospholipid is phosphatidyl choline (lecithin) and a surge in its production occurs at around 35 weeks' gestation in normal pregnancy, promoted by glucocorticoids. Fetal lung maturity seems to be accelerated in some cases of pre-eclampsia, growth retardation and premature rupture of the membranes and is delayed in diabetes mellitus. α-fetoprotein is of no relevance to pulmonary maturity.

27. B C E

The cystadenoma, granulosa cell tumour and teratoma may all occur in the ovary, being derived from neoplastic growth in epithelial, sex cord and germ cell structures, respectively. The nephroblastoma and neuroblastoma are developmental tumours of kidney and nerve tissue, respectively, occurring almost exclusively in early childhood and generally showing a sarcomatous appearance.

28. E

Amniocentesis, if performed under ultrasound guidance, is associated with a pregnancy loss of about 1:200. It does not appear that the position of the placenta increases the risk of placental wastage. Amniocentesis is useful to diagnose genetic disease and it is the ultrasound scan that is the diagnostic for open neural tube defects. It is interesting that 2% of amniotic fluid samples fail to culture and these have a higher association with a congenital abnormality.

29. A C

Chlamydia, although it has an intra-cellular existence, differs from a virus by its large size, complex cellular envelope and possession of both RNA and DNA. The treatment of choice is tetracycline, such as doxycycline, but if the woman is pregnant then erythromycin should be used. The common heat-stable antigen may be used as an enzyme-linked method of detection. *Chlamydia* may also be detected by direct staining smears. Fitzhugh–Curtis syndrome is a syndrome of fibrinous perihepatitis associated with pelvic peritonitis. The patient may present with upper abdominal pain and tubal damage can occur. Therefore, infertility is a long-term sequel.

30. A B E

- Postpartum haemorrhage (PPH) is a potentially life-threatening complication of both vaginal and Caesarean delivery. PPH is defined as blood loss greater than 500 ml during delivery. PPH can be divided into

  a. Primary PPH that occurs within 24 hours after delivery.
  b. Secondary PPH that occurs 24 hours to six weeks after delivery.

  The exact incidence of PPH is difficult to determine. PPH occurs in 2–8% of deliveries. Secondary PPH occurs in approximately 1% of all deliveries.

- The most frequent cause of PPH is uterine atony (90%) other causes include: lacerations of the cervix and/or vagina, retained placenta, disorders of coagulation and thrombocytopenia, uterine inversion and rupture uterus.

- Risk factors include the following: prolonged labour, pre-eclampsia, previous PPH, multiple gestation, coagulation abnormalities, forceps or ventouse delivery, multiparity (20–fold increase in risk) and polyhydramnios.

31. A C D E

Nausea and vomiting are the most frequent and perhaps the most troublesome symptoms of early pregnancy. The exact aetiology is unknown and the condition is usually self-limiting. Antihistamines are better than a placebo and are generally considered to be safe during pregnancy. Sometimes antihistamines can cause troublesome side-effects, including drowsiness and blurring of vision. It is important to remember that epigastric pain and late onset of nausea and vomiting may be a presenting feature of pre-eclampsia and, specifically, the HELLP syndrome. Increased trophoblastic tissue with a hydatidiform mole may give exaggerated signs of pregnancy; this may be not only excessive nausea and vomiting but also early pre-eclampsia. It is important that in the management of a patient with nausea and vomiting an ultrasound scan is performed.

32. All True

Chromosome abnormalities, particularly of the X chromosome, can occur. X-chromosome mosaicisms are the most common abnormality. In Turner's syndrome (45XO) accelerated follicular loss causes ovarian failure.

Familial premature ovarian failure has been associated with fragile X permutations. Women with Down's syndrome also have premature menopause.

Autoimmune diseases including hypothyroidism, Addison's disease and diabetes may be associated with premature ovarian failure.

The metabolic disease galactosaemia is associated with premature ovarian failure.

Hysterectomy with conservation of the ovaries can induce ovarian failure. In these women it is advisable to perform annual follicle-stimulating hormone measurements, especially in women who have had a hysterectomy before the age of 40.

Infection, including mumps and tuberculosis, may be associated with premature ovarian failure.

33. B D E

Basal body temperature measurement is a poor method for ovulation detection and has a very limited role (if any) in the investigation of an infertile woman. Basal body temperature often drops transiently by 0.1–0.2°C around the time of ovulation followed by a sustained rise of 0.5–1.0°C which is maintained throughout the luteal phase. The plasma luteinising hormone surges to a peak around 12 hours before ovulation and falls progressively during the luteal phase. Plasma progesterone secretion by the corpus luteum increases to a peak around 7–8 days after ovulation and, as a result, the endometrium undergoes a secretory change and cervical mucus becomes more scanty, viscid and cellular.

34. A C D

With antepartum haemorrhage, the patient requires hospital assessment and vaginal examination should not be performed until the placental site is known. In placental abruption, vaginal blood loss is not an accurate indication of severity.

35. E

In order to counsel a patient for sterilisation the acronym FILMVE should be used. The following must be ascertained:

F That the patient knows the failure rate is about 1:500

I That the patient has been fully informed that it is irreversible. If a patient thinks it is reversible then it is contraindicated.

L That the patient is aware that it is done by the laparoscopic method, although it may be necessary to do a mini-laparotomy if the tubes are not visible.

M That the patient knows that the menses should not be affected; however, if the patient has been on the pill before being sterilised then coming off the pill may be associated with heavy periods which is endogenous rather than exogenous in relation.

V That the partner has thought about a vasectomy.

E Ectopic

36. A D

With increasing maternal age there is an increase in chromosomal abnormalities associated with the increasing age of the oocytes. There is also an increase in the background luteinising hormone. Both of the above may predispose to an increase in miscarriage.

37. B C D

Genital herpes is usually caused by herpes virus hominis Type II, whereas ordinary lip herpes is caused by herpes virus hominis Type I. Penicillin and other treponemicidal drugs should NOT be given as they may confuse the diagnosis of coincidental syphilis.

38. A D E

Female sterilisation is the most commonly used method of contraception in the age group 40–49 years. Vasectomy is more popular in younger couples.

Healthy, normal body mass index, non-smoking women with no cardiovascular risk factors may continue to use the low-dose combined oral contraceptive pill until the age of 50 years. Women who smoke are best advised to stop at the age of 35 years.

The progestogen-only pill is an excellent form of contraception for the older woman as it has few contraindications, and is highly effective in this group if taken in the correct way. Poor cycle control is a major disadvantage.

Emergency contraception can be used in this group. The only contraindication being migraine at presentation in a woman with a history of migraine with aura. The progestogen-only method has been shown to cause less nausea and vomiting than the combined method and to have improved efficacy.

39. A B

Definitions of this type can cause difficulties as many books give subtly different answers.

Primary amenorrhoea is defined as no menstruation by 14 years of age with growth failure or absence of secondary sexual characteristics, ie breast development and pubic hair growth; or no menstruation by 16 years of age when growth and sexual development are normal.

Secondary amenorrhoea is defined as the absence of menses for six months in a previously menstruating woman.

The climacteric is the time when a woman changes from being able to sexually reproduce to being unable to sexually reproduce and puberty is the opposite, ie the time when a woman becomes able to sexually reproduce. The last menstrual period is the menopause and the first menstrual period is the menarche.

Dysmenorrhoea can be primary or secondary. Primary dysmenorrhoea is defined as pain which begins on the first day of menstruation but improves as menstruation proceeds. It usually occurs in the younger woman and is associated with ovulation. Secondary dysmenorrhoea is pain beginning 1–5 days before the onset of menstruation which is relieved by menstruation. It is usually associated with pathology in the older woman. Such pathology includes endometriosis, fibroids and pelvic inflammatory disease. It may also be associated with the intrauterine contraceptive device.

40. B D

Thrombosis and thromboembolism remain the **main direct cause** of maternal death. Although they account for 33% of all direct maternal deaths, the rate has fallen since the last Report.

Hypertensive disease of pregnancy remains the second leading cause of direct deaths, as it was in the last triennium. Like other leading causes of direct deaths the rate of maternal death has fallen compared to the last Report.

Sepsis, including deaths in early pregnancy following miscarriage and ectopic pregnancy, is the third leading cause of direct deaths. The rate of maternal deaths from sepsis is slowly increasing.

Taken as a whole, deaths in early pregnancy are the second leading cause of direct deaths. The deaths included in this group occur from several causes. The largest number is due to ectopic pregnancy (the fourth leading cause of direct deaths). **The Confidential Enquiries into Maternal Deaths in the United Kingdom (1997–1999), Executive Summary and Key Recommendations, RCOG website.**

41. A D E

There are three interrelated indications for the use of low-dose aspirin in pregnancy:

- For pre-eclampsia prophylaxis this is limited at present to those who are judged to be at risk of early onset of pre-eclampsia.
- Management of primary antiphospholipid syndrome which is associated with an increased risk of first- and second-trimester fetal loss, but also when at risk of thromboembolism, not only venous but also arterial.
- Thromboprophylaxis, although at present no randomised control study has been performed to confirm this.

42. A B C D

Gardnerella vaginalis is a Gram-negative bacillus. It is associated with bacterial vaginosis. Diagnosis can be difficult, but is aided by the following points:

- there is a disagreeable, fishy smell, particularly after intercourse
- clue cells which are bacteria attached to the vaginal epithelial cells are present
- the vaginal pH is >5: this is associated with both *Gardnerella* and *Trichomonas*

Gardnerella can be transported on Stuart's medium.

43. A B C D

Women who develop thrush post antibiotic therapy should be given anti-thrush agents prophylactically. Aqueous creams can be used as a soap substitute as well as an emollient for the vulval skin. Several studies have shown the effectiveness of maintenance therapy with antifungals once an induction regime has effected a cure.

Maintenance therapy for up to six months includes:

Fluconazole	100 mg weekly
Itraconazole	50–100 mg per day
Ketoconazole	100 mg per day
Clotrimazole	*per vaginam* weekly

Resistant yeasts can be treated with vaginal boric acid 600 mg daily for 14 days or topical flucytosine. Injections of medroxyprogesterone acetate have been used.

44. A C D E

Routine ultrasonography is beneficial to confirm gestational age early on and to look for congenital abnormalities between 16 and 20 weeks. The role of nuchal fold thickness scanning is being evaluated at present and has its uses as a screening test for Down's syndrome. Although the ultrasound scan is very helpful in the management of pregnancy, including the confirmation of dates, and the detection of twins, blighted ovum and hydatidiform mole, it is yet to reduce perinatal deaths not due to congenital abnormalities.

45. E

Puerperal psychosis usually begins within the first 7–10 days of the puerperium and most often takes the form of depression. Schizophrenia or mania are rare. The onset is often acute and the eventual outcome good. The risk of recurrence in subsequent pregnancies is between 1:3 and 1:7.

46. B D E

Fetal growth and size are very difficult to assess. The measurement by abdominal palpation is extremely crude and some people would even describe it as a blind guess. Clinically, the most widely practised techniques are measurement of the fundal height and of the abdominal girth at the level of the umbilicus. Several studies have demonstrated good sensitivity and specificity of fundal height for detecting low birth weight for gestation. It is, therefore, a useful screening test which can detect growth retardation. Maternal weight gain is of limited importance. Ultrasound is generally considered to be the best available method of measuring fetal size and growth.

47. B D E

During this triennium there have been significant decreases in deaths from pulmonary embolism and sepsis following Caesarean section. This is because of the routine introduction and use of guidelines which were introduced as a result of the recommendations from previous CEMD Reports (1994–96).

For the first time in this report (1997–99), the number of indirect deaths, due to pre-existing disease aggravated by pregnancy, is greater than deaths directly related to pregnancy.

The CEMD started to report deaths from mental illnesses in depth in the last triennial Report. However, when all deaths up to one year from delivery are taken into account, the results of the study show that deaths from suicide are not only the leading cause of indirect death, but also the leading cause of maternal deaths overall.

During 1997–99, 378 deaths were reported by the Enquiry, similar to the 376 cases reported in 1994–96. **The Confidential Enquiries into Maternal Deaths in the United Kingdom (1997–99), Executive Summary and Key Recommendations, RCOG website.**

48. A E

The incidence of preterm rupture of membranes (PROM) is approximately 10% of pregnancies. The terminology can be confusing. PROM is rupture of the membranes (ROM) prior to the onset of labour in a patient who is beyond 37 weeks' gestation. Preterm premature rupture of the membranes (PPROM) is ROM prior to the onset of labour in a patient who is less than 37 weeks' gestation. Patients with PROM may present with the chief complaints of leaking fluid and vaginal discharge. PPROM is associated with 30% of preterm deliveries, not PROM. Several studies have reported that, expectant management decreased the Caesarean delivery rate and length of labour without increasing the infection rate, especially in cases with an unfavourable cervix. The patient's desires should always be considered and the management options should be discussed with her, with careful documentation.

49. All true

Epidural analgesia is the most effective method of analgesia in labour. It often slows the second stage by reducing or eliminating the normal surge of oxytocin and by reducing pelvic floor muscle tone. This may lead to more instrumental deliveries.

A mixture of nitrous oxide and oxygen is one of the most common methods of obstetric analgesia that maintains consciousness. 'Entonox' is a 50:50 mixture of the two gases and acts on the central nervous system, resulting initially in analgesia and later in anaesthesia. Entonox takes 30 seconds to act and its effect continues for approximately 60 seconds after inhalation has ceased.

Transcutaneous nerve stimulation (TENS) produces electrical stimulation and provides a distraction while simultaneously gating the pain impulses at the level of the spinal cord.

Pethidine is a central nervous system depressant. This drug has an onset of action of about 15 minutes and a duration of action of 2–4 hours. A standard dose is 50–100 mg intramuscularly, repeated 1–3 hours later if necessary.

50. A D

Breast-feeding, compared with artificial feeding, has been clearly shown to protect against gastrointestinal infection in the infant and against necrotising enterocolitis among babies born at more than 30 weeks' gestation. Combined oestrogen–progestogen oral contraceptives should be avoided during breast-feeding as they could increase the incidence of breast-feeding failure. Oestrogen should not be used for lactation suppression as it increases the risk of vaginal bleeding and of thromboembolism.

For those who have lost a baby pharmacological suppression of lactation may be considered: bromocriptine is effective in lactation suppression but rebound lactation is common. Carbergoline, compared with bromocriptine, is more effective and may be used as a single dose.

In simple breast engorgement, antibiotics and oxytocin are unlikely to be beneficial. Unrestricted access for the baby to the breast still appears to be the most effective way to prevent and treat breast engorgement.

51. C D E

Dietary advice should focus on a well-balanced and varied diet with adequate daily folate, iron, calcium (1200 mg) and fluids (2–3L). Foods likely to be infected with Listeria should be avoided, e.g. raw meat, raw seafood and soft cheeses.

Exercise is commonly restricted to non-contact sports after 16 weeks. Ideally, vigorous exercise should be limited to 15–20 minutes.

There are good data to show that pelvic floor exercise undertaken antenatally results in stronger pelvic floor muscles postnatally and this may have an influence on continence status and genital prolapse in the future.

Problems may arise at different times during pregnancy, so the assessment for risk factors and complications must be an ongoing process throughout pregnancy, labour, delivery and the postpartum period. Some women will require more visits than others. A minimum of four antenatal visits is recommended for a woman with a normal pregnancy (Antenatal Care Report of a Technical Working Group, 1994 – WHO).

52. B D

A pruritus vulva is the term given to itching affecting the genital area of women. It should be distinguished from vulvodynia, which refers to chronic burning symptoms. Skin conditions such as dermatitis, psoriasis, or lichen sclerosis CAN CAUSE PRURITUS VULVAE. At least 10% of women all over the world suffer from this complaint. One of the main causes of pruritus vulvae is purulent and mucopurulent vaginal discharge. Over 80% of cases have this cause. Glycosuria and diabetes also contribute to this condition.

53. A C E

The International Society for the Study of Vulvovaginal Disease (ISSVD) defines vulvodynia as chronic vulval discomfort or pain. Characterised by itching, burning, stinging, or stabbing in a vulva in which there is no infection or skin disease of the vulva or vagina. The pain can be unprovoked, varying from constant to intermittent. This condition is also known as vulvar vestibulitis syndrome or vestibulodynia. Often the vagina shows no abnormalities or signs of infection. Unfortunately, many doctors are unaware of this condition and may suggest to their patients that it is a psychological condition.

54. A B

For uncomplicated pregnancy, induction of labour with vaginal prostaglandin agents can be conducted on antenatal wards. However, women with recognised risk factors (including suspected fetal growth retardation or previous Caesarean section), the induction process should not occur on an antenatal ward.

Wherever induction of labour occurs, facilities should be available for continuous fetal heart rate monitoring. Cardiotocography should be established immediately prior to induction of labour. Prolonged use of maternal facial oxygen therapy may be harmful to the fetus and should be avoided. Where oxytocin is being used for induction or augmentation of labour, continuous electronic fetal monitoring should be used.

55. C D

Physical signs suggestive of early pregnancy include changes in the breasts and Hegar's sign, a softening of the cervical isthmus occurring around six weeks' gestation. Physical signs during the first trimester are unreliable predictors of pregnancy (low sensitivity).

The average duration of pregnancy is 266 days from the date of ovulation. If calculation is made according to the first day of the last menstrual period, the average duration is 280 days. Ovulation most frequently occurs on the 14th day of a 28-day cycle.

Uterine enlargement commences shortly after implantation and four weeks after conception, the rate of enlargement is approximately 1 cm per week. Fifty per cent of pregnant women will experience nausea and vomiting between two weeks and 12 weeks after conception.

56. C D

Fertilisation of the human ovum occurs in the lateral or ampullary part of the uterine tube approximately 12–24 hours after ovulation, and the ovum then passes along the tube to the cavity of the uterus where implantation occurs approximately 5–7 days after fertilisation. Fertilisation comprises the union of the spermatozoon with the mature ovum. Under normal conditions only one spermatozoon enters the ovum and takes part in the process of fertilisation. Spermatogenesis occurs in the seminiferous tubules of the testes and begins at puberty.

57. A B E

Trophoblastic cells produce human chorionic gonadotrophin (hCG). Serum levels of this hormone rise steadily during the first six weeks of pregnancy. During this early stage of pregnancy, hCG levels double every 1.3–2 days.

Modern urine pregnancy tests can detect hCG concentrations as low as 25 mIU/mL; 98% of women will have positive urinary pregnancy test by seven days after implantation.

Radioimmunoassay techniques for measuring concentrations of serum β-hCG can detect levels as low as 2–10 mIU/mL.

58. All True

The following are all risk factors for ectopic pregnancy:

Previous history of pelvic inflammatory disease or other pelvic infection: *Chlamydia* and *Gonorrhoea* are both able to grow within the Fallopian tubes and cause damage to the endosalpinx, and peri-tubal adhesions. Other pelvic infections, such as appendicitis, can also result in pelvic adhesions and thus increase the ectopic pregnancy rate.

Previous tubal surgery: such as reversed sterilisation with tubal re-anastomosis, micro-surgery for infertility and unexpected pregnancy after sterilisation.

Previous history of ectopic pregnancy: there is a roughly 10-fold increase in ectopic pregnancy.

Intrauterine contraceptive device (IUCD) *in situ*: all but the progesterone-containing IUCDs are relatively protective against ectopic pregnancy while the IUCD is in place. That is, the number of ectopic pregnancies in women using an IUCD for contraception is about one-half that in women using no contraception. However, when IUCD pregnancies occur there is a greater chance of an ectopic location (3–4%).

Assisted conception technology (*in vitro* fertilisation and gamete intrafallopian transfer): the risk of a heterotopic pregnancy (previously thought to be 1 per 30000 pregnancies) increased significantly in women conceiving with one of the assisted reproductive technologies (up to 1 per 100 pregnancies).

A history of diethylstilboestrol exposure *in utero*. There are often uterine cavity defects that may limit intrauterine implantation. Also, tubal defects exist that may increase the chance for a tubal ectopic pregnancy.

59. A B C E

Human chorionic gonadotrophin (hCG) is detectable in the blood or urine 1–2 days after implantation (10 days after ovulation). It increases rapidly (doubling every 36–48 hours in the first six weeks), reaching a peak 60–80 days after fertilisation; then drops off quickly to 10–30% of the peak value for the rest of the pregnancy. It serves to maintain progesterone production by the corpus luteum in the early part of pregnancy, and also stimulates the development of the fetal gonads and synthesis of androgens. At levels of 1000–1500 IU/L, an intrauterine sac should normally be seen using transvaginal ultrasound.

60. All True

The incidence of cord prolapse is 0.14–0.62% with a perinatal mortality between 8.6–49%. There are several recognised risk factors:

- abnormal presentation (breech, transverse lie and oblique lie)
- high parity
- high presenting part
- multiple pregnancy
- pelvic tumours
- pre-term rupture of membranes
- polyhydramnios
- prematurity and/or low birth weight

OSCE
Practice Exams

The Objective Structured Clinical Examination

Introduction

The Objective Structured Clinical Examination (OSCE) for the DRCOG was introduced in the Autumn 1994 examination. It now replaces the oral and viva sections of the exam.

A series of preset tasks, clinical problems, or other test situations are set up and the candidate moves around them at timed intervals. Marks for performance at each station are awarded according to a previously agreed schedule.

There are several advantages to this method. As the same 'station' is experienced by each candidate there is fairness in the examination. The candidate is directly observed at work on the task without the intrusive influence of the examiner. Certain areas of competence can be specifically tested. The marking system has been tested to ensure that candidates are marked consistently.

Practical aspects of the OSCE examination for the DRCOG

1. Carefully note the place and correct time to arrive at your examination centre. Arrive with plenty of time to spare.
2. You will be sent an entrance card before the examination. On your entrance card is the station number at which you start.
3. There is a 'holding area' and in this area there will be a plan of the examination stations and a sample question for you to inspect.
4. The stations are laid out in a clockwise direction 1–22.
5. When directed by the invigilator, proceed to your designated station.
6. Each OSCE has a circuit of 22 stations or tables. Of these, two are rest stations and 20 are active stations. You may actually start with a rest station.
7. Each station will have:
   - A card indicating the number of the station.
   - An answer book with your name and candidate number on it. You MUST check that these match the candidate number on your College entrance card. If not, inform a member of staff.
   - Examination material which will be face down.

8. Open your answer book until the station number shown in the top right hand corner of the page matches the number of the station where you are.
9. When the bell rings (one long ring), turn over the examination material and start. YOU MUST READ THE QUESTIONS CAREFULLY.
10. You have six minutes at each station.
11. On each answer sheet there are boxes for your answers. Your answer must be confined to the appropriate box any other writing on the sheet will not be considered by the examiners. Thus, brief answers are appropriate.
12. At the end of six minutes, two rings of the bell signify that your time is up.
13. With this bell:
    - Stop.
    - Leave your answer sheet in the tray provided.
    - Proceed as directed to the next station.
    - Sit down and commence the next task.
    - Make sure you have your answer booklet open at the new station number.
14. No textbooks, calculators, or similar articles are allowed.
15. No form of communication between candidates during the examination is allowed.
16. Candidates are not permitted to copy any part of the OSCE paper.
17. All OSCE questions must be answered. Failure to respond clearly to every question may result in loss of marks.
18. Candidates must stop writing when told to do so. Continuing to write after each station has ended will result in a substantial loss of marks.
19. No candidate is allowed to leave during the examination.
20. Smoking is not allowed.
21. Raise your hand if you wish to attract the attention of the invigilator.

Exam centre areas

Reception area ↓	Welcome to candidates
Holding area	Plan of examination stations Refreshments Registration Briefing
Marshalling area ↓	45 minutes before the examination
OSCE circuit	

This arrangement allows two examinations to be held on the same day.

The OSCE stations

The OSCE has a circuit of 22 stations or tables, of which two are rest stations and 20 are active stations. All OSCE questions are created by a consultant, discussed at a committee and piloted before they eventually enter the bank of questions.

Each station is marked out of 10 and the different designs include:

- Factual stations. These test different aspects of knowledge and problem solving to those tested by the MCQ paper. The OSCE question may ask you to *'Give three possible differential diagnoses...'* There may be eight actual answers. Sometimes drugs are mentioned and they may ask about dosage and route. X-rays, photographs, partograms and so on may be presented.
- Task orientated stations. These involve carrying out a task, eg *'Test this urine sample.'*
- Communication stations. Role players are used here. It is vital to introduce yourself and to ascertain to whom you are speaking! Scenarios could include:
  - Candidate to patient explaining how to take the pill.
  - Candidate to midwife discussing a case of suspected growth retardation.
  - Candidate to GP explaining the history behind a stillbirth.
  - Candidate to consultant discussing a case of a pelvic mass.
  - Candidate to husband explaining that the patient (his wife) has ovarian carcinoma.

Marks could be awarded for:
  - Introducing yourself.
  - Putting the patient at ease.
  - Explaining the condition.
  - Not using too much medical terminology, if talking to a non-medical person.
  - Following verbal clues.
  - Following non-verbal clues.

The role player may also give marks for:
  - Good eye contact.
  - Being a listening doctor.
  - Providing confidence.
  - *'I would like to see this candidate again'*

- Structured orals. Candidates will be given written information about which they will be asked structured questions. Ten marks are awarded and the examiner has a marking scheme against which he works. An example of such a structured oral would be:

You are a hospital doctor and a GP (the examiner) is about to see a patient who has a prolapse of the uterus. What advice can you give the GP before he sees the patient as to what investigations can be done and what medical and surgical treatments can be offered?

The structured oral and communication stations are interactive. They are like a well-structured viva but perhaps a little artificial. There are approximately five interactive stations in the circuit.

OSCE Practice Exam Instructions

To obtain maximum benefit from the following 40 questions, restrict yourself to a maximum of six minutes for each question, allowing a total of two hours for each paper. Either write your answers in the boxes provided or use a separate sheet of paper. (In the exam, answer sheets with boxes to write in will be A4 in size.)

Remember, there may be many possible answers to each question and you may be asked to write only one or two of these answers. You will gain no marks from writing more answers than are requested. One-word or short note answers are acceptable.

The explanatory notes at the end of this section are comprehensive and include correct answers to every question.

OSCE Practice Exam 1

20 stations: time allowed 2 hours (6 minutes per station)

1

Caroline S is a 19-year-old student. She comes to your surgery complaining of an altered vaginal discharge. She is obviously very embarrassed about this and seeks your confidential help.

1. What three questions may help you make the diagnosis? (3 marks)

2. On examination you find a grey, mucoid discharge which has a slightly fishy smell. What is the likely diagnosis? (1 mark)

3. What simple office test would help you to confirm this diagnosis? (1 mark)

4.   What treatment would you give for the above condition? (1 mark)

5.   Give two other common infectious causes of vaginal discharge and appropriate treatments in each case. (2 marks)

Cause
Treatment
Cause
Treatment

6.   List two non-infectious pathological causes of vaginal discharge. (2 marks)

2

A 35-year-old woman is eight weeks pregnant for the first time. She has no serious past medical history and neither she nor her partner have a history of any serious congenital abnormality. She is keen to have counselling about her risks for Down's syndrome.

1. What are her age-related risks of having a Down's syndrome baby at term? (1 mark)

| |
| |

2. What two screening tests could she be offered and at what gestation? (4 marks)

Screening Test
Gestation
Screening Test
Gestation

3. What two diagnostic tests can be offered and what are their associated miscarriage risks? (4 marks)

Diagnostic Test
Miscarriage Risk
Diagnostic Test
Miscarriage Risk

4. What diagnostic test can be done to exclude neural tube defects? (1 mark)

3

The following smear result is obtained:

ST ELSEWHERE HOSPITAL BORCHESTER	
Name: Mrs A.J.	Date: 26.2.95
LMP: 5.2.95	Date of Birth: 20.3.63
Cervical smear demonstrating severe dyskaryosis.	

1.   Give two actions you will take. (2 marks)

2.   At colposcopy the following is detected:

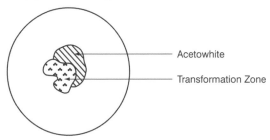

Acetowhite

Transformation Zone

Give two treatments appropriate to the above colposcopic findings
(2 marks)

3. Give two short-term risks of these treatments. (2 marks)

4. List two specific pieces of advice you would give to your patient before the procedure. (2 marks)

5. The histology comes back as severe dyskaryosis and you are happy that complete excision has been performed. What follow-up is required over the next five years? (2 marks)

4

Andrew is a 27-year-old car mechanic who smokes 20 cigarettes a day and enjoys a night out in the pub at the weekend. He needs to be investigated for infertility. Examination is found to be normal. You ask for a semen sample for analysis.

1. What advice would you give to him about collection of the semen sample? (2 marks)

2. The following results come back from the laboratory:

Volume   3 ml
Count 14×10^6/ml
Motility   20% actively motile 10% sluggishly motile
            70% non-motile
Morphology 70% look abnormal

Give one normal and two abnormal findings from this result. (3 marks)

Normal	
Abnormal	
Abnormal	

3. Knowing the above history, list two pieces of advice that you should offer him. (2 marks)

    +---+
    | |
    | |
    +---+
    | |
    | |
    +---+

4. Four months later two repeat semen analyses are reported as normal. His wife is ovulating and has regular periods. They have now been trying for 20 months. Indicate with a 'yes' or 'no' what actions you would consider appropriate:

    • to keep trying naturally for another six months YES/NO (1 mark)
    • perform a diagnostic laparoscopy and dye   YES/NO (1 mark)
    • *in vitro* fertilisation   YES/NO (1 mark)

5

You have been asked to see a lady in her first pregnancy at 27 weeks' gestation, who has had a significant exposure to chickenpox whilst the contact was infectious. A careful history confirmed that this lady is not immune to Varicella Zoster virus (VZV) and she has had a significant exposure just four days ago.

1. What would you offer her? (2 marks)

2. What are the fetal risks/complications? (2 marks)

3. What are the maternal risks/complications? Name two (2 marks)

4. When would you refer her to the hospital? Name four referral criteria (1 mark)

You have been asked to see a lady, 25 weeks pregnant, who presented with suspected first-episode genital herpes.

5. How would you manage her infection? (2 marks)

6. How would you deliver her? (1 mark)

6

You have been asked to counsel a lady, who is 14 weeks pregnant and is a heavy consumer of alcohol. A careful history confirms that she consumes approximately 18 units of alcoholic drink per day.

1. Fetal alcohol syndrome is a rare event but is a serious complication of heavy alcohol consumption during pregnancy. What is the risk of incidence of this syndrome in this particular patient? What are the characteristic features of this syndrome? Name two features (2 marks)

2. Women should be careful about alcohol consumption in pregnancy. What is the maximum recommended limit of alcohol during pregnancy? (1 mark)

You have been asked to see a woman who is 26 weeks pregnant, who complains of left leg discomfort with tenderness. Clinical examination shows swelling, tenderness, increased temperature and oedema. You suspect deep vein thrombosis.

3. What would you do for her? List two diagnostic tests to confirm your diagnosis. (3 marks)

The diagnostic test is negative but a high level of clinical suspicion still exists.

4. What would you do next? (2 marks)

You have been asked to see an eight weeks pregnant woman who smokes 15–20 cigarettes/day.

5. What are the effects of heavy smoking in her pregnancy? Give four possible complications? (2 marks)

7

Mrs T. Z. is a 47-year-old lady who presents to your surgery complaining of hot flushes and superficial dyspareunia. Her last period was five months ago. She is using the intrauterine device for contraception.

1. From the above history, what is the most likely diagnosis? (1 mark)

2. What blood test will help to confirm this diagnosis? (1 mark)

3. She is keen to try hormone replacement therapy for this problem. Give two different routes of administration of oestrogen. (2 marks)

4. If you were to give unopposed oestrogen, what is the patient at increased risk of developing? (1 mark)

5. Give two long-term benefits of hormone replacement therapy. (2 marks)

6. Give two contraindications for hormone replacement therapy. (2 marks)

7. Six months after going onto hormone replacement therapy her follicle-stimulating hormone level is found to be 34 IU/l. What advice can you give her regarding contraception? (1 mark)

8

Miss X. K. is a 25-year-old P0+0. Her last period was five weeks ago. She presents to you with mild left iliac fossa pain for the past three days associated with mild vaginal bleeding for one day. Her transvaginal scan shows the following:

Transvaginal scan performed

Anteverted uterus with thickened endometrium measuring 14.4 mm.

Right ovary appears normal. Left ovary surrounded by cystic area which has the ultrasonic appearance of hydrosalpinx.

No free fluid seen.

No evidence of ectopic on the scan but I cannot exclude this.

Reported by Senior Radiographer.

---

1. Give four differential diagnoses for the left-sided lesion? (4 marks)

Miss W. M. is a 32-year-old (P2+0). Her last menstrual period was 10 weeks ago. She presents to you with brownish vaginal discharge for eight days. Her transvaginal scan shows:

> *Transabdominal and Transvaginal scans performed.*
>
> *Single fetus of crown rump length 17 mm seen in utero.*
> *No fetal heartbeat detected.*
> *Appearances are that of a missed miscarriage, fetal demise occurring at approximately 8 weeks, 2 days.*
> *Patient referred to EPC.*
>
> *Reported by Senior Radiographer.*

2. What is your diagnosis? (1 mark)

3. How would you manage Miss W. M.? Give three options. (3 marks)

Read the following scan and answer question 4.

> Two gestation sacs in retroverted uterus.
> Fetal poles seen × 2.
> Fetal heartbeat detected × 2.
> Crown rump length × 2 = 8 mm = 6+ weeks = dates.
> EDD 6/11/03
> Ovaries appear normal. No free fluid seen.
>
> Reviewed and electronically signed by Senior Radiographer.

4. What is the incidence of this type of pregnancy? Give two predisposing factors for this type of pregnancy? (2 marks)

9

A 25-year-old primigravida is admitted in labour at 38 weeks' gestation.

Her cervix is 4 cm dilated and the fetal membranes are intact. She is having two contractions every 10 minutes, which are described as strong and lasting for 30 seconds.

Four hours later, her cervix is 5 cm. Her midwife decides to perform artificial rupture of membrane (ARM) to enhance the labour.

1. Name three contraindications in general for ARM? (3 marks)

2. Name two complications for ARM. (2 marks)

Two hours later, her contractions are infrequent and short lasting.

3. What would be your next step? (1 mark)

Four hours later (after regular and strong contractions), her cervix is still 5 cm dilated.

4.   Name two possible causes.(3 marks)

```
┌─────────────────────────────────────┐
│                                     │
│                                     │
├─────────────────────────────────────┤
│                                     │
│                                     │
└─────────────────────────────────────┘
```

The registrar on call performed a vaginal examination, which shows head –3, cervix still 5 cm dilated, large caput and moulding.

5.   What would you do next? (1 mark)

```
┌─────────────────────────────────────┐
│                                     │
│                                     │
│                                     │
└─────────────────────────────────────┘
```

10

Mrs P. J., aged 32, stopped taking the combined oral contraceptive nine months ago. Since then she has had no periods and is anxious to know why.

1. Fill in the table below concerning the history of this condition. (NB You must consider three different diagnoses.) (6 marks)

Question asked in history	Diagnosis you are considering
a.	d.
b.	e.
c.	f.

2. List three useful blood tests to help make the diagnosis. (3 marks)

3. Mrs P. J. wants to conceive. What are the chances if, after treatment, ovulation is induced? (1 mark)

11

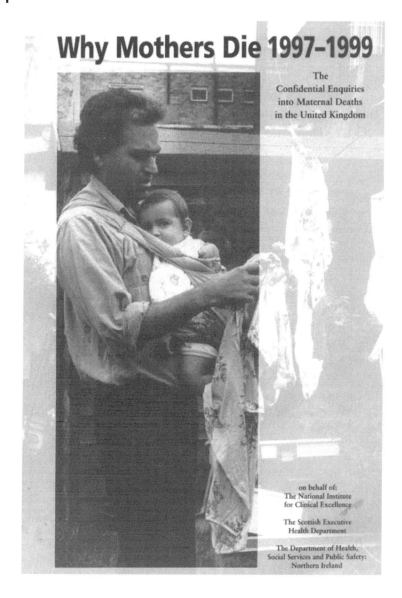

Above is the cover of a book called *Why Mothers Die 1997–1999* (RCOG Press, 2001).

1. What is the other name of this report? When was the first report published? (2 marks)

2. The report summarises the causes of maternal mortality into three main categories. What are they? (3 marks)

3. What is the maternal mortality rate in this triennium (1997–1999)? (2 marks)

4.   What are the commonest two causes for maternal death in the UK?
     (2 marks)

5.   What is the leading cause of maternal death in early pregnancy in
     the UK? (1 mark)

12

Read the following referral letter:

Dear Doctor

I would be grateful if you could see Mrs H. B. who is pregnant again. This is her sixth pregnancy having had a termination of pregnancy in 1990, normal delivery of Mike in 1992, a daughter Linda born in 1994 by Caesarean section but unfortunately died at 12 days because of complication of surgery for jejunal atresia, second son Peter was born by Caesarean section in 1996 and she had a daughter Nicola born in 2001 by elective Caesarean section.

She has had problems with varicose veins during pregnancy and a history of asthma which exacerbated during her last pregnancy.

Her last period was on 10 July this year, giving her an estimated delivery date around 25 April next year. Although this pregnancy was not planned, she is happy to be pregnant again.

Yours truly,

Dr Evans

---

1. List four risk factors for her current pregnancy. (2 marks)

2. What is the effect of the pregnancy on her asthma? (1 mark)

3. What is the effect of the uncontrolled asthma in her pregnancy? Give three complications. (3 marks)

4. What could this patient do to relieve the discomfort from her varicose veins? Give four pieces of general advice. (2 marks)

5.   What is the incidence of jejunal atresia? What is the chance of this recurring in this pregnancy? (2 marks)

13

This question relates to family planning.

1.   Complete the table below. (6 marks)

Methods of contraception with a failure rate of <1 per 100 woman years	Methods of contraception with a failure rate of 2–3 per 100 woman years	Methods of contraception with a failure rate of >10 per 100 woman years
a	c	e
b	d	f

2.   Give two methods that can be used as emergency contraception and their failure rates. (4 marks)

Method	Failure rate
a	
b	

14

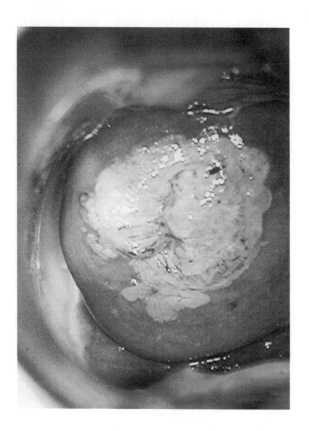

1. Look at the photograph and list three differential diagnoses.
    (3 marks)

2. How would you confirm diagnosis? (1 mark)

3. List three referral criteria to the colposcopy clinic. (3 marks)

4. The pathology result comes back as CINIII. What is the treatment of choice? What are the possible complications? List two complications. (2 marks)

5. How would you follow this patient after her treatment? (1 mark)

15

Mrs R. J. is a 24-year-old bank clerk. She is eight weeks pregnant and is complaining of severe nausea and vomiting. You examine her abdomen and the fundus is compatible with a 14-week uterus.

1.   Give three differential diagnoses. (3 marks)

2.   List three investigations you would organise. (3 marks)

3.   The scan demonstrates a molar pregnancy. What is the treatment of choice? (1 mark)

4. What follow-up is arranged? (2 marks)

5. What advice would you offer for future family planning? (1 mark)

16

You are a hospital doctor who received the following referral letter:

Dear Doctor

I would be grateful for your help with Mrs K, who is 26-years-old and has been suffering with vaginal spotting after intercourse as well as irregular vaginal bleeding between her periods for the last six months.

Her previous cervical smear two years ago was normal. She is using the combined pill for contraception. Mrs K is otherwise fit and well.

Yours truly,

Dr Smith

---

1. List four causes for her bleeding. (3 marks)

Clinical examination shows a healthy-looking cervix, uterus normal size anteverted, mobile and both adnexa were free.

2.   List three useful investigations for her bleeding. (3 marks)

In another patient with a similar history, speculum examination shows a cervical ectropion.

4. Name two common situations where you would find cervical ectropion. (2 marks)

5. Give two possible treatment methods for a cervical eversion? (2 marks)

17

Interpret the following results:

Mrs Jackson, a 32-year-old old patient, presents to you with history of primary sub-fertility for five years. Her blood result is shown below:

Progesterone	
Day in cycle	*22*
Progesterone	*54.2 nmol/L*

1. What is the significance of this result? (2 marks)

Mr Jackson is 36 years old and in good health, he has no children from any previous relationships. His semen analysis result is shown below:

SPECIMEN(S):	*Infertility semen*
VOLUME:	*3 ml of fluid*
COUNT:	*170 million per ml*
MOTILITY:	*40% motile, 10% sluggish,*
	10% non-progressive, 40% non-motile
CYTOLOGY:	*3% normal, 97% abnormal forms*
DR KJ	

2.   Name any abnormalities in Mr Jackson's semen result? (2 marks)

3.   It was decided that Mr Jackson needs to repeat the semen analysis test again in a few weeks. Give Mr Jackson three essential pieces of advice regarding his semen collection. (3 marks)

The second semen result comes back as a normal.

4.   What is your next investigative step regarding Mr and Mrs Jackson's sub-fertility? Name three different investigation methods appropriate for this step. (3 marks)

18

These two instruments are commonly used in labour ward.

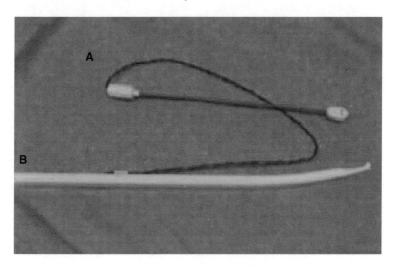

1.   What are the names of these instruments? (2 marks)

A
B

2.   Give three reasons to use device B? (3 marks)

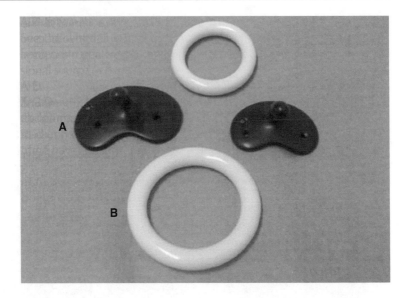

3. These devices are commonly used in gynaecology outpatient clinics. What are they? (2 marks)

A	
B	

4. Give three reasons (indications) to use device B in patients with genital prolapse. (3 marks)

19

Below is a recording of a normal cardiotocograph (CTG).

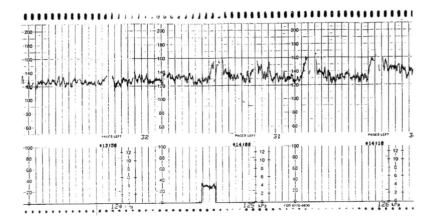

1. List three good markers about the CTG. (3 marks)

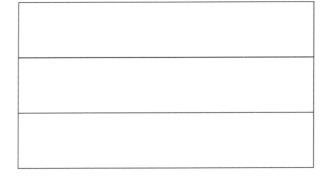

Below is a recording of an abnormal CTG of a woman not in labour.

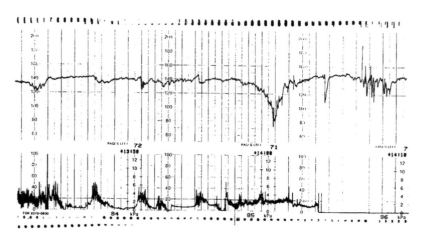

2.   List two reasons why this is abnormal. (2 marks)

| |
| |
| |

3.   What other test can be performed in labour to assess the wellbeing of the baby and give the normal level? (2 marks)

| *Test* |
| |
| *Normal Level* |

4.   At what level would immediate delivery be required? (1 mark)

| |

5. What other evidence in labour may indicate fetal compromise and why? (2 marks)

20

Read the following referral letter:

> Dear Doctor
>
> I would be grateful for your help with Miss Y who has been suffering bouts of perineal and lower pelvic pain since January last year.
>
> She continues to suffer episodes of pain and has also noted that she has more severe pain after intercourse and that pain is worse during her period. Throughout the last two months she has had no change in her bowel habits and does not suffer pain on defecation. She continues to pass urine normally.
>
> On examination there was some tenderness of her loaded sigmoid colon but no rebound abdominal tenderness. Vaginal examination revealed severe pain caused by moving the cervix.
>
> She has been referred to Mr X (surgeon) at the nearest hospital for sigmoidoscopy, but I wonder whether she needs further gynaecological investigation.
>
> Yours truly,

1. List three important questions to identify the cause of her pain. (3 marks)

2. What are the possible gynaecological causes of her chronic pelvic pain? List three causes. (3 marks)

You have decided to perform diagnostic laparoscopy to identify the source of her pain.

3. What are the indications for diagnostic laparoscopy for chronic pelvic pain? (1 mark)

4. What is the incidence of negative diagnostic laparoscopy (no significant pathology) for chronic pelvic pain? (1 mark)

5. All your investigations come back as a normal and no obvious organic causes for her pain. How would you treat her? Give two options. (2 marks)

OSCE Practice Exam 1:
Answers and Teaching Notes

1

Normal vaginal secretions consist of desquamated epithelial cells, vaginal wall transudate, mucus from the cervix, some material from the upper genital tract and micro-organisms.

Doderlein's lactobacilli are the most prominent bacteria. This produces the normal acidic vaginal pH and this mechanism helps resist pathogenic infection.

A cyclical variation in vaginal discharge is also common.

Important questions raised by the history include the symptom of pruritus. A recent change in sexual partner is significant as this would increase one's suspicion of a sexually transmitted organism. Diabetes or immunosuppression is associated with *Candida*. It is also important to take a good contraceptive history. If the patient has recently changed the pill, then there may be a hormonal cause and the introduction of latex, etc. may indicate an allergy. Any of these would be a good answer to the first part of this question.

The type of discharge detected at the speculum examination is important. A foreign body can sometimes be detected and this may present with a bloodstained, foul smelling discharge. *Candida* gives a white creamy non-odorous discharge. Bacterial vaginosis produces a grey mucoid discharge with a fishy smell. Bacterial vaginosis is associated with a vaginal pH above 4.5. This is the office test that could be done. *Trichomonas* is associated with a yellow-green discharge and strawberry haemorrhages on the cervix. Pelvic inflammatory disease is associated with a purulent cervical discharge accompanied by other signs of systemic infection including a temperature and pelvic tenderness.

Bacterial vaginosis is treated with 400 mg of metronidazole twice daily for five days or clindamycin vaginal cream.

Candida can be treated by clotrimazole or fluconazole. Patients should also be advised to take simple measures, such as wearing loose cotton underwear and avoiding irritants such as bath additives.

Trichomonas is treated by 2 mg of metronidazole stat. or 400 mg of metronidazole twice daily for five days. It is also important to trace sexual partners and search for other sexually transmitted diseases.

Other causes of cervical infections include *Neisseria gonorrhoeae* and *Chlamydia trachomatis*.

There are many non-infectious pathological causes and these include foreign body, chemical vaginitis, neoplasia of the cervix or vagina, vaginal prolapse or fistula, and cervical eversion.

It is important not to forget physiological causes of vaginal discharge and these include puberty, the menstrual cycle, sexual activity, pregnancy and the menopause.

2

The age-related risk of having a Down's syndrome child at 35 years of age can be seen from the table below:

Risk of Down's syndrome at delivery

Age	Risk	Age	Risk	Age	Risk
20	1:1923	30	1:835	40	1:109
21	1:1695	31	1:826	41	1:85
22	1:1538	32	1:725	42	1:67
23	1:1408	33	1:592	43	1:53
24	1:1299	34	1:465	44	1:41
25	1:1205	35	1:365	45	1:32
26	1:1124	36	1:287	46	1:25
27	1:1053	37	1:225	47	1:20
28	1:990	38	1:177	48	1:16
29	1:935	39	1:139	49	1:12

Remember that the risks are greater during the first trimester and there is then a natural loss towards term.

It is very important to distinguish between screening tests and diagnostic tests. Screening tests ((a) nuchal fold thickness scanning, (b) triple blood test) only give you a risks ratio; they are not diagnostic.

Nuchal fold thickness scanning can be done at 11–14 weeks' gestation. The triple blood test, which includes the measurement of α-fetoprotein, oestriol and β human chorionic gonadotrophin, is perhaps more widely used and is offered at 14–16 weeks.

Diagnostic tests ((a) amniocentesis, (b) chorionic villus sampling) carry a miscarriage risk. An amniocentesis, which is done at 16 weeks, has an associated miscarriage risk of approximately 1:200, whereas a chorionic villus sample, which is done after 11 weeks, has a miscarriage risk of approximately 1:20.

Open neural tube defects are screened for in some units by performing an α-fetoprotein test, but the diagnosis is now made by detailed scanning.

3

This smear demonstrates moderate dyskaryosis which is a cytological diagnosis compatible with the diagnosis of severe dysplasia. The two actions
that are most important are to explain the situation carefully to the patient
and to arrange for her to have a diagnostic colposcopy. You should clearly
state what the problem is and especially indicate that this is evidence of
premalignant and not malignant disease. There are potentially a lot of
psychosexual complications following this and, therefore, careful counselling is important. As the upper limit of the transformation zone was
clearly seen at colposcopy, local out-patient therapy is possible. The
different forms of treatment include:

- Large loop excision of the transformation zone. This is probably the
  preferred treatment as a large amount of tissue is made available to
  the histopathologist without destruction.

- A laser cone. This is done in some units and has the same advantage
  as a large loop excision.

- Cold coagulation of the cervix.

- Laser ablation of the cervix.

The last two are suitable treatments, but do run into the problem that only
the biopsy demonstrates the pathology; a larger sample of tissue may
indicate a different pathology and, therefore, a potentially different
follow-up.

There are several short-term risks of treatment and these include infection
and bleeding. The specific advice that should be given to your patient can
be demonstrated by the acronym THIS. This stands for:

T do not use Tampons, but pads for the next four weeks
H if you have any heavy bleeding (Haemorrhage) heavier than a period
   when you are not expecting a period then it is important to contact
   your General Practitioner
I avoid Intercourse for the next four weeks
S if Sultrin cream has been advised, this should be given for the next
   10 days on a nightly basis

The routine follow-up after adequate treatment is to have a smear 6 and
12 months post-procedure and then annually for five years. Assuming
these are all negative then the patient can go back to a routine recall for a
smear every three years.

4

The general advice for a patient who is required to produce a semen sample for analysis is to abstain from ejaculation for a maximum of five days and a minimum of three days before the sample is produced. Therefore, if a patient was due to give a sample on a Thursday, he should have intercourse for the last time on the Sunday. It is important for the sample to be brought immediately to the laboratory. Ideally, it should be produced on-site.

The semen analysis result demonstrates oligoteratoasthenospermia, ie a low sperm count, poor motility and morphology. The volume was normal.

The general advice that he should be given is to cut down or stop smoking as well as to stop 'binge' drinking.

It would be very reasonable for the couple to keep trying for another six months without any further treatment or investigations. As his wife is ovulating and Andrew's semen analysis has returned to normal, to continue trying is the treatment of choice. It would be reasonable to do a laparoscopy and dye in order to assess tubal patency. With unexplained subfertility in a couple who have only been trying for 20 months, *in vitro* fertilisation would be inappropriate in this age group.

5

The answers to this question come from the RCOG Clinical Green Top guidelines.

If the pregnant woman is not immune to varicella zoster virus (VZV) and she has had a significant exposure, she should be given VZ immunoglobulin (VZIG) as soon as possible. VZIG is effective when given up to 10 days after contact. Women who have had exposure to chickenpox (regardless of whether or not they have received VZIG) should be asked to notify their doctor or midwife early if a rash develops.

Maternal infection after 20 weeks and up to 36 weeks does not appear to be associated with adverse fetal effect but may present as shingles in the first few years of infant life.

Although varicella infection is much less common in adults than in children, it is associated with greater morbidity, namely pneumonia, hepatitis and encephalitis.

Indications for referral to hospital include the development of chest symptoms, neurological symptoms, haemorrhagic rash or bleeding, a dense rash with or without mucosal lesions and significant immunosuppression. If the woman smokes cigarettes, has chronic lung disease, is taking steroids, or is in the latter half of pregnancy, hospital assessment should be considered, even in the absence of complications.

Any woman with suspected first-episode genital herpes should be referred to a genitourinary clinic. Treatment with acyclovir should be considered for all women who develop a first episode of genital herpes in pregnancy and a screen for other sexually transmitted infectious diseases should be arranged.

Vaginal delivery is recommended (if there is no contraindication) for this patient who develops first episode genital herpes lesions during the first or second trimesters and no active lesion during labour. However, Caesarean section is recommended for all women presenting with first episode genital herpes lesions at the time of delivery.

6

The answers to this question come from the RCOG Clinical Green Top guidelines.

The syndrome is not seen consistently in infants born to women who are heavy consumers of alcohol and occurs only in approximately 30–33% of children born to women who drank about 2 g/kg of body weight per day (equivalent to approximately 18 units of alcoholic drink per day).The diagnosis of fetal alcohol syndrome requires signs in all of the three following categories:

- Fetal growth restriction.

- Central nervous system involvement (neurological abnormalities, developmental delay, intellectual impairment, head circumference below the third centile, brain malformation).

- Characteristic facial deformity (short palpebral fissures, elongated mid-face, flattened maxilla)

During pregnancy, women should limit their alcohol consumption to no more than one standard drink per day. One unit of alcohol approximately equals 8 g of absolute alcohol, which is equivalent to:

- ½ pint of ordinary strength beer, lager, or cider

- ¼ pint of strong beer or lager

- 1 small glass wine

- 1 single measure of spirits

- 1 small glass sherry

In women with factors consistent with venous thromboembolism, anticoagulant treatment should be employed until an objective diagnosis is made. Some of these symptoms and signs are commonly found in normal pregnancy. Diagnostic imaging should be performed promptly in pregnant women with suspected deep vein thrombosis (ultrasound or X-ray venography). In pregnancy, D-dimer can be elevated due to the physiological changes in the coagulation system and particularly if there is a concomitant problem such as pre-eclampsia. Thus a 'positive' D-dimer test in pregnancy is not necessarily consistent with venous thromboembolism and objective diagnostic testing is required.

If ultrasound is negative and a high level of clinical suspicion exists, the patient should be anticoagulated and ultrasound should be repeated in one week. X-ray venography should be considered. If repeat testing is negative, anticoagulant treatment should be discontinued.

Smoking during pregnancy is estimated to account for 30% of low-birth-weight babies (1.8–2.4 times greater risk of having a lower birth weight baby), up to 14% of preterm deliveries, and some 10% of all infant deaths (20% increase in perinatal mortality if the mother smokes more than 20 cigarettes/day). Also there is increased risk of vaginal bleeding and 1.5 times greater risk of spontaneous miscarriage. Smoking can decrease quality and quantity of breast milk by 30%. Maternal smoking during and after pregnancy has been linked to asthma among infants and young children. Cigarette smoking in the first trimester was associated with a small increased risk of having a child with a cleft lip/palate and a child with isolated cleft.

7

Mrs T. Z. is probably menopausal. The menopause is strictly defined as one day in a woman's life, ie the last period. The time during which a woman changes from being able to sexually reproduce to being unable to sexually reproduce is called the climacteric.

The blood test which helps to confirm the diagnosis is for follicle-stimulating hormone; a result persistently above 20 IU/l is diagnostic of ovarian failure.

Hormone replacement therapy can now be given by several routes. These include tablet, patch, gel and hormone implant.

The main risk of giving unopposed oestrogen is that of endometrial hyperplasia leading to endometrial carcinoma. Studies have indicated that there is a 6% incidence of endometrial carcinoma after five years of unopposed oestrogen and 20% after 10 years of unopposed oestrogen. To prevent endometrial hyperplasia, cyclical progestogens are used in order to change proliferative to secretory endometrium and then shed it with a period. A progestogen causes a withdrawal bleed on an oestrogen-primed endometrium.

The benefits of hormone replacement therapy include prevention of typical menopausal symptoms, such as hot flushes, night sweats and insomnia, but the long-term benefits are that of the prevention of osteoporosis and possible cardiovascular disease.

Minimum bone-sparing doses of oestrogen given daily are:

Conjugated equine oestrogens	0.625 mg
Oestradiol valerate	1 mg
Transdermal oestradiol	50 μg
Oestradiol implants	25 mg

Epidemiological studies suggest a 50% reduction in osteoporotic fracture with five years' use of hormone replacement therapy.

Oestrogen therapy is effective in reducing cardiovascular and cerebrovascular disease in postmenopausal women. Therapy benefits not only the lipid profile but also insulin metabolism and the myocardial and cerebral blood flows.

Breast cancer, endometrial cancer and undiagnosed irregular vaginal bleeding, active liver disease are contraindications to hormone replacement therapy.

With a follicle-stimulating hormone level of 34 IU/l, Mrs T. Z. will be postmenopausal. As she may be under 50, it is probably best to advise her to

173

continue to use the intrauterine contraceptive device (IUCD) for one year, ie one year after her last bleed (to be certain of not conceiving).

In the box you should write 'Keep the IUCD in place until one year has passed since her last natural period'. As it is impossible when on hormone replacement therapy to state when her last natural period was, you have to assume that her last period before the blood test was a natural one.

8

The top priority in this situation is to determine whether or not this patient is pregnant. This can be done simply by positive pregnancy test or measurement of serum β human chorionic gonadotrophin level. Adnexal masses include a wide spectrum of disease entities from an extension of physiological changes to highly malignant ovarian neoplasm. The differential diagnosis will include ectopic pregnancy, benign parovarian cysts, localised abscess and hydrosalpinx, corpus luteum cyst (common in first 16 weeks of pregnancy), benign ovarian cyst and ovarian neoplasm.

Missed miscarriage (presence of a non-viable fetus). In this condition there is either failure of embryonic growth (blighted ovum) or the viable fetus dies. Recommended alternatives which may be used for both include silent miscarriage, delayed miscarriage, or early fetal demise.

The majority of women with missed miscarriage are referred to hospital for assessment and up to 88% currently undergo surgical uterine evacuation using suction curettage. 'Medical evacuation' and 'expectant management' are accepted alternative techniques, although they have not replaced surgical evacuation. Both mifepristone (RU 486) and misoprostol have been used to empty the uterus.

Twin births over the past decade have risen by 33%. Twin pregnancies occur at a rate of 1:85 pregnancies in the UK, 80% are dizygotic twins. Monozygotic twinning occurs at a relatively constant rate of 3–5 in 1000 births world-wide. Factors associated with dizygotic twins:

- Multiparity > 3.

- Clomiphene therapy (up to 7–17% incidence).

- Gonadotrophin therapy (up to 18–50% incidence).

- Increased maternal age.

- Race: common in Nigeria (dizygotic twinning, occurs from 1:1000 births in Japan to nearly 50:1000 births in parts of Nigeria).

- Family history of twins (maternal side).

Twin pregnancy is a mixed blessing. Maternal adaptations to pregnancy are exaggerated with twins. In the first trimester all the physiological changes seen in singleton pregnancy occur to a greater degree (nausea, vomiting, anaemia), also spontaneous miscarriage is three time greater than singleton pregnancy. Twin fetuses are at very high risk for the increased morbidity and mortality that accompany premature delivery and congenital anomalies, both of which occur more commonly in the twin pregnancy. Polyhydramnios, placental abruption, placenta praevia, pre-eclampsia occur more often in twin pregnancy.

9

Intact fetal membranes have been described as the biggest single hindrance to progress in labour and clearly artificial rupture of membrane (ARM) has a potent labour-promoting effect. In general the following could be considered as a contraindication for ARM:

- Malpresentations such as transverse lie, footling breech
- Active herpetic lesions in the vulva or vagina
- Vaginitis or cervicitis (eg group β streptococci, until antibiotic prophylaxis has been initiated)
- Human immunodeficiency virus
- Hepatitis B
- Unstable presentation.

ARM carries two particular hazards. Firstly, in the absence of a well-fitting presenting part, the umbilical cord may prolapse. Secondly, pathogenic bacteria may be introduced, especially if delivery is delayed.

Start her on oxytocin: oxytocin is of little clinical value prior to ARM. Oxytocin can be employed immediately after the ARM or its use may be delayed until the response to membrane rupture is assessed.

During the active phase of labour the cervix should dilate at a rate of at least 1 cm/hour, if not then failure to progress in labour is diagnosed. When the partogram indicates that the progress in labour is suboptimal the simplest method of establishing the cause is to identify which of the three components (namely the powers, passenger, or the passages) are responsible.

- Poor uterine contraction
- Malposition, usually occipitoposterior
- Malpresentations
- Large baby
- Deficient pelvis (uncommon).

Caesarean section.

10

It is not the oral contraceptive pill that has caused the problem and it would have occurred in this individual anyway.

This is a case of secondary amenorrhoea and differentials include:

- Premature ovarian failure in which case the woman will be complaining of hot flushes and night sweats and other menopausal symptoms.

- Polycystic ovarian syndrome the patient will be complaining of hirsutism, acne, or increasing weight.

- Hyperprolactinaemia may be a cause and this could be secondary to anti-psychotic drugs or a micro- or macro-adenoma of the pituitary.

- One must always exclude a pregnancy and it is important to the history to ask about symptoms of pregnancy, such as nausea, vomiting, or fetal movement.

- Anorexia can be associated with amenorrhoea and, therefore, it is important to assess recent weight changes.

- Hypothalamic causes include hypogonadotrophic hypogonadism and this could be associated with Kallmann's syndrome which can be associated with loss of smell.

- Excessive exercise

From the above, appropriate answers to Question 1 would include:

- Any hot flushes or night sweats – premature ovarian failure

- Any milk coming from breasts – hyperprolactinaemia

- Any symptoms of pregnancy

- Any weight loss – anorexia

Diagnosis can be made by assessing follicle-stimulating and luteinising hormones and oestradiol, which can help diagnose not only polycystic ovarian syndrome but also hypogonadotrophic hypogonadism and premature ovarian failure.

Prolactin levels are useful for the assessment of hyperprolactinaemia and a urinary pregnancy test may well be useful.

Conception in these cases is very good once ovulation has been stimulated and drugs that can be used for this include clomiphene citrate and human menopausal gonadotrophin which need to be given by injection. The answer to Question 3 is 'Good' or 'A little below that for the normal population'. A multiple pregnancy is a potential side-effect of this treatment.

11

This booklet summarises the key findings and recommendations made in the **Fifth Report of the Confidential Enquiries into Maternal Deaths (CEMD) in the United Kingdom 1997–1999**. The key messages it contains are of relevance to all commissioners of maternity care and health professionals who plan or care for women during or after their pregnancy. These include GPs, midwives, obstetricians, staff in Emergency Departments, psychiatrists, anaesthetists and pathologists. The first report was published in 1952.

The Enquiry includes deaths directly related to pregnancy (Direct), those due to pre-existing disease aggravated by pregnancy (Indirect), those in which the cause was unrelated to pregnancy (Coincidently, previously identified as Fortuitous).

During this triennium 378 deaths were reported to or identified by the Enquiry, a number remarkably similar to the 376 cases reported in 1994–96. Overall maternal mortality rates (Direct and Indirect deaths) known both to the Registrars General and to this Enquiry. The maternal mortality rate for this triennium, derived from the CEMD data, is 11.4 deaths per 100 000 maternities. The Direct maternal mortality rate is 5.0 deaths per 100 000 maternities. The Indirect maternal mortality rate is 6.4 deaths per 100 000 maternities.

Thrombosis and thromboembolism remain the major direct cause of maternal death. They account for 33% of all direct maternal deaths. Hypertensive disease of pregnancy remains the second leading cause of direct deaths.

Ectopic pregnancy is the leading cause of maternal death in early pregnancy in the UK.

12

A high-risk pregnancy is any pregnancy that puts either the mother or the fetus at risk. Classifying pregnancy as low or high risk is an effective way to deliver extra attention to the patient who needs extra care. All pregnancies should be carefully evaluated to identify any risk factors. This particular patient is grand multi-gravid who had three previous Caesarean sections, history of neonatal death due to congenital abnormality, history of bad asthma in her last pregnancy and problems with her varicose veins.

In general, one-third of women have a decline in their asthma status, one-third have improved, and one-third remain unchanged during pregnancy. Some women with severe asthma may develop high blood pressure or pre-eclampsia during pregnancy. There is an increased risk of having a low-birth-weight baby or a preterm delivery in women with uncontrolled asthma. Asthma is very rarely a problem during labour.

When asthma is controlled, women with asthma have no more complications during pregnancy and labour than non-asthmatic women. Induction of labour with prostaglandin E2 is safe. Ergometrine, which can cause a severe attack theoretically, should be avoided for the active third stage. Syntocinon, on the other hand, is effective and safe. If a Caesarean is necessary, epidural or spinal is better than a general anaesthetic, to reduce the chance of chest infection. There are no problems with breast-feeding whilst taking any of the asthma treatments.

Approximately 40% of all pregnant women suffer from varicose veins. There are several reasons for this including increased blood volume, and increased levels of progesterone. The following advices can help to minimise the discomfort of pregnancy-related varicose veins such as:

- Avoid standing for long periods of time

- Mild exercise, such as walking

- Wear compression stockings

- Avoid excessive weight gain during pregnancy

- Elevate the legs at the end of the day

Intestinal obstruction is found in about 1 per 2000 births. The condition is usually sporadic. Associated chromosomal defects are rare. Diagnosis of obstruction is usually made quite late in pregnancy (after 25 weeks) by ultrasound (jejunal and ileal obstructions are imaged as multiple fluid-filled loops of bowel in the abdomen). The chance of jejunal abresia recurring is less than 1%.

13

The failure rate per 100 woman years equals:

$$\frac{Total\ number\ of\ pregnancies}{1200} \times Total\ months\ use$$

Methods that are very effective (failure rate of <1 per 100 woman years) include sterilisation, either of the man or woman, the combined oral contraceptive pill, or depo-progestogen injections.

Methods that are slightly less successful, but still effective (failure rate in the order of 2–3 per 100 woman years) include the progestogen-only pill, the intrauterine contraceptive device, the diaphragm or cap with a spermicide or the condom with spermicide.

Less effective methods (failure rate in the order of 10 per 100 woman years) include spermicide alone and the contraceptive sponge. Coitus interruptus also has a failure rate of this order.

Anybody who requires emergency contraception should be counselled according to their long-term contraceptive needs.

The two emergency contraception methods that are available are the hormonal method and insertion of the coil.

Hormonal emergency contraception now involves the use of Levonorgestrel. It is effective if the first dose is taken within 72 hours of unprotected intercourse. Taking the first dose as soon as possible increases efficacy.

Levonorgestrel may be used 72–120 hours after unprotected intercourse but this is an unlicensed use, but efficacy decreases with time.

Levonorgestrel is taken as one tablet of 750 mg followed 12 hours later by a further tablet. If vomiting occurs within three hours of taking the tablet, a replacement dose can be taken. If an anti-emetic is required, Domperidone is preferred.

Many centres would recommend routine follow-up of all postcoital patients for future contraception and to exclude pregnancy.

Insertion of the coil is an effective method if fitted within five days of exposure to unprotected intercourse. Obviously, it is difficult in cases of rape or nulliparity because there is a greater risk of sexually transmitted infection. This method is 95% effective, although a previous ectopic pregnancy is a contraindication.

14

This is a focal abnormal colposcopy appearance after the application of acetic acid. It is the most commonly found of all abnormal features associated with the abnormal transformation zone, but is not diagnostic of cervical intraepithelial neoplasia (CIN). It might be found associated with human papillomavirus infection, immature squamous metaplasia, leukoplakia, CIN and microinvasion cervical carcinoma.

It is important that the colposcopist detects the abnormal colposcopic appearance of premalignant conditions. Appearance of these conditions can be confusing. Biopsy of an area of doubt is the only way to confirm the diagnosis.

- Moderate and severe dyskaryosis

- Any suspicious looking cervix even if the smear is negative

- Worrying symptoms such as postcoital bleeding

- Cervical cancer is found occasionally in women with postmenopausal bleeding

- Persistent mild dyskaryosis, persistent inflammatory smears or inadequate smears

In the UK, large loop excision of transformation zoon (LLETZ) is the treatment of choice. Many other types of treatment are available and they can be divided into two groups. Firstly excisional methods where the transformation zoon is removed intact, and secondly destructive or ablative methods.

Pain and haemorrhage and infection are the possible complications. Significant haemorrhage is quite uncommon (less than 2% of all cases). Secondary haemorrhage can occur any time up to 14 days and is usually the result of a minor infection. This occurs in 1–2% of treated women. Cervical stenosis is much more likely to occur after large conaization and affected 1–2% of women managed by LLETZ.

A typical follow up protocol would be as follows:

- Colposcopy clinic in six months for Colposcopy and cytology assessment

- Annual smear from 12 months to five years after treatment. Thereafter women would return to routine recall.

Follow up is essential for any Colposcopy management. The reasons are:

- Ensure no residual CIN
- Detect any recurrence of CIN
- Ensure no clinical problem since treatment

15

The differential diagnosis of this case is:

- Hydatidiform mole
- Twin pregnancy
- Wrong dates

In order to assess the large fundus an ultrasound scan is the investigation of choice.

In order to investigate the nausea and vomiting a good history and examination are needed. Check the maternal urea and electrolytes and liver function as well as the urine in order to exclude a urinary tract infection. Severe cases of hyperemesis gravidarum require admission, intravenous hydration and occasionally anti-emetics.

In this case a molar pregnancy has been detected.

Molar pregnancies occur in approximately 1:2000 women in the UK, but in Asians they occur in up to 1:200 pregnancies. The aetiology is unknown, but complete moles contain 46 chromosomes of paternal origin and may lead to choriocarcinoma. Partial moles, which are more common, have 69 chromosomes with the additional set coming from paternal origin.

The treatment of choice is a suction evacuation. Sometimes prostaglandins are required if the uterus is thought to be too large for surgical evacuation and in older women a hysterectomy is considered.

Follow-up is monitored by measuring the β human chorionic gonadotrophin (βhCG) and referral to a regional centre; these are in London (Charing Cross Hospital), Sheffield and Aberdeen.

Appropriate short answers to Question 4 would be:

- Refer to a regional centre
- Monitor hCG

hCG follow-up will range from six months to two years after evacuation of the hydatidiform mole.

Initially, serum samples are requested and, once these have returned to normal, urine samples are requested. If the patient's hCG values return to normal within eight weeks of evacuation, follow-up is usually limited to six months. Patients in this group need not be further delayed in starting a new pregnancy.

Patients who do not have normal hCG values within eight weeks of evacuation should have a 2-year follow-up. In this group it is reasonable to allow a patient to try for a further pregnancy after the hCG has been normal for six months. In this group the risk of choriocarcinoma occurring after hCG has been normal for six months is 1:286.

Further estimates of hCG 6 and 10 weeks after any future pregnancies are requested because of the small risk of choriocarcinoma developing in these patients.

Hormonal preparations for contraception or other purposes, taken between the evacuation of the mole and the return to normal of the hCG values appear to increase the risk of invasive mole or choriocarcinoma developing. It is recommended that these preparations should be avoided until the hCG has become undetectable in the serum.

A good short answer to Question 5 would be 'Avoid pregnancy and use non-hormonal methods of contraception until advised by regional centre'.

16

Postcoital bleeding (bleeding after intercourse) is more likely to originate from the vagina or cervix than the endometrium. Intermenstrual bleeding is defined as bleeding from the vagina at any time in the menstrual cycle other than normal menstruation.

Causes (postcoital and intermenstrual bleeding) include:

- Infections: vaginitis and/or cervicitis
- Cervical carcinoma and, very rarely, vaginal carcinoma
- Cervical polyps
- Cervical ectropion
- Trauma

Additional causes for intermenstrual bleeding include:

- Contraceptive pill causing breakthrough bleeding
- Intrauterine contraceptive device
- Progestogen-only pill
- Contraceptive injection, eg Depo-Provera
- Miscarriage – especially in a young woman
- Pregnancy test should be considered
- Cervical smear if not done yet
- Transvaginal ultrasound
- Hysteroscopy and endometrial biopsy

An ectropian describes the situation in which columnar epithelium replaces the stratified squamous epithelium that normally covers the vaginal portion of the cervix.

Ectropion is an oestrogen-dependent condition and is commonly seen in women taking combined oral contraceptive pills, during pregnancy and after miscarriages. It also occurs in newborn infants and may persist into childhood.

Troublesome erosion may be treated by:

- Diathermy cauterisation
- Cryosurgery
- Laser treatment

17

This test confirms ovulation. In women with regular periods the most reliable method to confirm ovulation is to measure **midluteal phase serum progesterone level**. Ovulation is indicated by progesterone level equal or greater than 30 mmol/l.

Mr Jackson's semen result shows teratozoospermia: this is reduced levels of normally shaped sperm (<15% sperm of normal morphology). WHO guidelines (1999) recommend that a sperm sample showing 15% or more sperm of normal morphology should be considered normal.

All semen samples should be obtained by masturbation into a clean wide-mouthed non-toxic plastic container. Coitus interruptus is not recommended as the first part of ejaculation (containing a greater density of sperm) may be lost. It is important to deliver the sample at body temperature and within one hour of collection. It is good practice to advise the male not to ejaculate for three days prior to collection. At least two specimens should be examined during the course of investigation.

At the second consultation review with the couple the result of semen analysis and the ovulation test. If the results are normal then they should proceed to assessment of tubal patency. Tubal patency may be assessed by:

- Diagnostic laparoscopy and dye test

- Hysterosalpingography – this is the instillation of a radiopaque dye through the cervix under radiographic control

- Salpingoscopy and falloposcopy – salpingoscopy is passing a very fine rigid endoscope through the fimbrial end of the tube during diagnostic laparoscopy procedure. Falloposcopy involves passing a fine flexible fibre optic device from the uterine cavity into the Fallopian tube.

18

a. A fetal scalp electrode is a device used to obtain a fetal electrocardiogram during labour and delivery. It establishes electrical contact between fetal skin and an external monitoring device by a shallow subcutaneous puncture of fetal scalp tissue.

b. Amnio hook (a long type hook, with a pricked end) is used for artificial rupture of membrane (ARM) during labour.

Three reasons to perform ARM during labour are:

- To induce or augment labour
- To check for meconium-stained liquor
- To place a fetal scalp electrode

Vaginal pessaries

a.   Shelf pessary

b.   Ring pessary

Genitourinary prolapse can be reduced with vaginal pessaries. Pessaries may be appropriate while the patient is awaiting definitive surgery and when surgery is declined or contraindicated because of pregnancy or for medical reasons

Indications for use of vaginal pessaries

- If patient is medically unfit for surgery
- To gain relief from symptoms while awaiting surgery
- If further pregnancies are planned
- During pregnancy

19

In answer to Question 1, the good markers shown are:

- Rate between 120 and 160

- Accelerations

- Good variability

A normal fetal heart rate is 120–160 bpm. Brief accelerations of up to 10–15 bpm indicate a healthy fetus and good variability should also be demonstrated on the cardiotocograph (CTG).

A tachycardia, ie a heart rate >160 bpm is associated with certain drugs, prematurity, hypoxia, or maternal pyrexia.

The baseline bradycardia, ie <120 bpm may be significant if there is deceleration, but in severe cases may be pre-terminal.

Loss of baseline variability may indicate chronic hypoxia.

Decelerations can be early, this is usually due to compression of the fetal head and is not a sign of fetal distress, or late and these are usually associated with fetal hypoxia. Variable decelerations are often very difficult to interpret, but may be associated with cord compression.

In answer to Question 2, two reasons why this CTG is abnormal are:

- Loss of variability

- unprovoked deceleration

Fetal blood sampling is useful when the fetal heart rate recording is abnormal. A pH of >7.25 is normal, between 7.2 and 7.25 is borderline and should be checked within 30–60 minutes, but anything less than 7.2 is abnormal and delivery should be performed immediately.

Meconium staining of the liquor is due to hypoxia which causes vagal stimulation of the gut, relaxing the sphincter. However, it is not a good indicator in prematurity because of immaturity of the autonomic nervous system. Thick fresh meconium is an ominous sign as is the absence of liquor. Bleeding would also concern you if it occurred in labour.

20

Chronic pelvic pain can be puzzling to both doctors and patients, because the pain can be caused by multiple, overlapping problems. History taking is essential in evaluating chronic pelvic pain and should emphasise certain areas.

To approach a patient with chronic pelvic pain you must take into account five major sources of the origin of this pain:

- Gynaecological
- Psychological
- Musculoskeletal
- Urological
- Gastrointestinal

By a very careful history and physical examination the cause of the pain may be determined and appropriate therapy provided.

History taking should emphasise on the following:

- Current symptoms: duration and frequency, location and severity of pain. Medications and therapies tried.
- Past medical and surgical history.
- Gynaecological history should include sexual activity, exposure to sexually transmitted diseases, age at menarche, menstrual irregularities, and gravidity and parity.
- Urinary symptoms: frequency, dysuria, or hematuria may suggest a urologic cause.
- Gastrointestinal symptoms: dietary history, nausea or vomiting, and bowel habits to evaluate gastrointestinal sources of pain.
- Psychosocial symptoms: history of depression, eating disorders or substance abuse.

A woman with chronic pelvic pain must undergo a systematic and thorough investigation in order to rule out a variety of conditions. Gynaecological conditions which can cause pelvic pain include:

- Infectious causes such as pelvic inflammatory disease or tubo-ovarian abscess

- Adnexal lesions, such as ovarian tumours
- Pelvic adhesions (controversial)
- Pelvic congestion syndrome
- Fibroids, a presumed cause of chronic pelvic pain and a common cause of hysterectomy, have never been proven to cause chronic pelvic pain.

Chronic pelvic pain is the reason for 10% of all office visits to a gynaecologist and for over 40% of laparoscopies performed by gynaecologists.

- Dysmenorrhoea after failed medication
- Suspected organic lesion
- Suspected pelvic inflammatory disease
- Suspected endometriosis.

In general, about 40% of the patients will have no apparent pathology at laparoscopy. Findings at time of laparoscopy varied, depending on patient selection, and preoperative suspicion of endometriosis.

Chronic pelvic pain with no apparent organic cause is best treated by a multidisciplinary approach which includes a gynaecologist, nutritionist, psychologist and other specialists as needed.

Reassurance and providing sympathy and support for the patient's symptoms and the family's concerns can provide a true therapeutic release to the patient's disease.

When all organic causes of pelvic pain have been ruled out, a psychological evaluation may be required. These women are much more likely to have been physically and sexually abused as children and adults.

The woman may benefit from advice from a nutritionist about a high-bulk diet and from evaluation for possible food irritants, such as milk. Physical therapy in the form of heat, ultrasound, whirlpools and exercises may be helpful adjuvant therapy for the lower back and hip muscles.

Medical therapy may include combined contraceptive pills and non-steroidal anti-inflammatory agents, danazol or gonadotrophin-releasing hormone agonists.

Finally, a hysterectomy can be successful in some women who have not responded to medical therapy. In studies of referral populations, 60–75% of women had significant improvement of pain after hysterectomy, and 25–40% continued to have chronic pelvic pain despite surgery.

OSCE Practice Exam 2

20 stations: time allowed 2 hours (6 minutes per station)

1

A pregnant woman (G2P1) presented to the maternity unit at 32 weeks' gestation with fresh mild vaginal bleeding. Her first pregnancy ended with Caesarean section for fetal distress in labour.

1. List four possible causes for her bleeding. (4 marks)

| |
| |
| |
| |

On examination the cardiotocograph was reactive. Her abdomen was soft, not tender, equal to 33 weeks' gestation, with cephalic presentation. Speculum examination showed normal looking closed cervix with mild bleeding. The SpR on call ordered a transvaginal ultrasound for her.

2. Is transvaginal ultrasound an appropriate investigation for her? Why? (2 marks)

The ultrasound report showed an anterior low-lying placenta 10 mm away from the internal cervical os.

3. Name a condition which might be associated with her previous obstetric history. (1 mark)

Five hours later the woman started to bleed heavily, the obstetric registrar on call decided to deliver the baby by an emergency Caesarean section.

4. What issues (name two) should be considered when obtaining her consent? (2 marks)

5. Who should be involved in her management? (1 mark)

2

Mrs P. T., a 37-year-old woman, presents to your surgery complaining of the recent onset of painful periods. They have been gradually getting worse over the last few years. She is otherwise well, and is on no medication.

1. Give two possible differential diagnoses. (2 marks)

2. Name two investigations that may be useful to help you make the diagnosis. (2 marks)

3. Give three possible medical treatments. (3 marks)

4. Her 15-year-old daughter, Hannah, is having a similar problem. What is the most probable underlying cause? (1 mark)

5. Name two drugs that her daughter may find useful. (2 marks)

3

Mr and Mrs A. J. have been married for five years. Joanna has been trying to get pregnant for the last year. She is a 26-year-old secretary whose last period was five months ago. She does not smoke and is otherwise well. Andrew is a 27-year-old car mechanic who smokes 20 cigarettes a day and enjoys a night out in the pub at weekends.

1. List three questions you would specifically ask Mrs A. J. following the above history. (3 marks)

2. The following blood results were obtained:

   Follicle-stimulating hormone   4.3 IU/litre
   Luteinising hormone   5.6 IU/litre
   Prolactin   2754 IU/litre

   What is the diagnosis? (1 mark)

3. Name one other investigation that you would now perform. (1 mark)

4. What two possible treatments can you give Joanna? (2 marks)

5. Joanna is commenced on medical treatment. Give two common side-effects of the drug used. (2 marks)

6. Joanna becomes pregnant. What advice about her drug therapy should you give? (1 mark)

4

A 31-year-old woman who is pregnant for the first time presents to your GP surgery at 36 weeks' gestation. She complains of some epigastric discomfort and has a blood pressure of 180/120. On testing, her urine has ++protein.

1. What will you do? (2 marks)

2. Name four tests which should be performed in hospital. (4 marks)

3. It is decided that she needs to be delivered. What needs to be done to help decide the route of delivery? (1 mark)

4. What blood test must be done prior to labour/delivery? (1 mark)

5. What method of pain relief should be offered for labour? (1 mark)

6. Postpartum, what needs to be watched carefully? (1 mark)

5

You have been asked to see the following patient:

Dear Doctor,

I'd be grateful for your help with this 74-year-old lady who has had an episode of postmenopausal bleeding. Unfortunately I was unable to perform a satisfactory vaginal examination due to discomfort on her part. She describes an episode of bright red vaginal spotting which occurred when she was on holiday. This settled and then she had an episode of brownish discharge which has continued. She feels well in herself otherwise.

On examination today the vaginal area appeared atrophic and it was virtually impossible to open the speculum to view the cervix. However, I could not feel any abnormality on a gentle bimanual examination.

Yours sincerely

Dr Smith

---

1.   Give three possible causes of postmenopausal bleeding? (3 marks)

Your physical examination was satisfactory and unremarkable. You organise for her to have a transvaginal scan.

2. What is the importance of a transvaginal scan in the investigation of postmenopausal bleeding? (2 marks)

Endometrial cancer may present in 10% of women with postmenopausal bleeding.

3. Give three factors which may increase the relative risk of endometrial cancer. (3 marks)

4. List two outpatient investigation methods (except ultrasound) for postmenopausal bleeding? (2 marks)

6

You have been asked to see the following patient:

> *Dear Doctor,*
>
> *Re: Mrs M. R.*
>
> *I'd be grateful if you would consider this 29-year-old lady for sterilisation. She has four children age range five years to six months and unfortunately she recently became pregnant again and needed a termination at 10 weeks' gestation.*
>
> *Her husband is undergoing some investigation with Dr N (physician) and therefore is currently not particularly suitable for surgery.*
>
> *She would be very grateful if you would consider her for laparoscopic sterilisation if appropriate.*
>
> *Yours truly,*
>
> *Dr Jones*

1. How would you counsel Mrs M. R. about laparoscopic sterilisation? Give four important issues to cover during your counselling. (4 marks)

2. Mrs M. R. asks you if her sterilisation can be reversed. And, if yes, what is the successful rate? (2 marks)

3. Mrs M. R. is using Microgynon 30 for contraception. She is anxious about her period and asks if her laparoscopic sterilisation will affect her menstruation. She also asks when she can stop her pills. (2 marks)

4. Would you organise any follow-up? Why? What would you advise her on discharge from the hospital? (2 marks)

7

Plotted by EDD _____
which was derived from
LMP of _____ / early scan.
(delete as appropriate)

Name _____
Hosp. No. _____
(or name label)

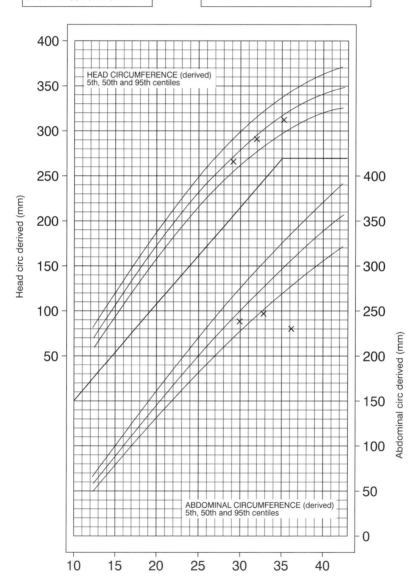

1. What is the name of this chart? What are the main components?
(3 marks)

2. What is the name of the abnormality?
(1 mark)

3. Name three methods for diagnosis and evaluation of this condition?
(3 marks)

4.   Name two maternal causes for this condition. (2 marks)

5.   What are the fetal risks associated with this condition? Give two
      fetal complications. (1 mark)

8

Congenital abnormalities are always a concern for the mother.

1. What blood screening test is available for an open neural tube defect? (1 mark)

2. What diagnostic test is available for an open neural tube defect? (1 mark)

3. What is the incidence of congenital heart defects? (1 mark)

4. What would make you consider congenital heart disease in the newborn? (3 marks)

5. What is the incidence of congenital dislocation of the hip (CDH)? (1 mark)

6. Which infants are more likely to develop CDH? (2 marks)

7. What is the incidence of phenylketonuria? (1 mark)

9

A 34-year-old woman is admitted to the ward at 36 weeks' gestation. She is unbooked and has recently passed about two cupfuls of fresh blood vaginally. She has some lower abdominal pain and tenderness and looks pale.

1. List the two most important differential diagnoses. (2 marks)

2. List two important actions you are going to take. (2 marks)

3. The pain and bleeding increase. How would you manage this case? (2 marks)

4. Postpartum she continues bleeding. What medical agents could be used to help stop the bleeding? (2 marks)

5. If the postpartum bleeding continues despite medical treatment what investigations are essential? (2 marks)

10

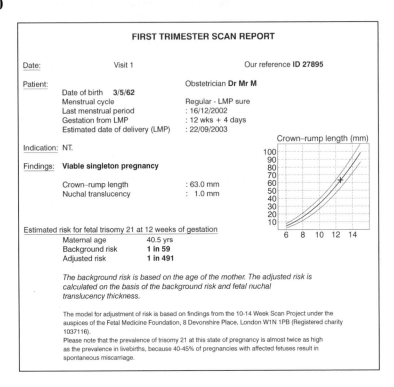

FIRST TRIMESTER SCAN REPORT

Date: Visit 1   Our reference **ID 27895**

Patient:

Date of birth   **3/5/62**
Menstrual cycle   Regular - LMP sure
Last menstrual period   : 16/12/2002
Gestation from LMP   : 12 wks + 4 days
Estimated date of delivery (LMP)   : 22/09/2003

Obstetrician **Dr Mr M**

Indication: NT.

Findings: **Viable singleton pregnancy**

Crown–rump length   : 63.0 mm
Nuchal translucency   : 1.0 mm

Crown–rump length (mm)

Estimated risk for fetal trisomy 21 at 12 weeks of gestation

Maternal age   40.5 yrs
Background risk   **1 in 59**
Adjusted risk   **1 in 491**

The background risk is based on the age of the mother. The adjusted risk is calculated on the basis of the background risk and fetal nuchal translucency thickness.

The model for adjustment of risk is based on findings from the 10-14 Week Scan Project under the auspices of the Fetal Medicine Foundation, 8 Devonshire Place, London W1N 1PB (Registered charity 1037116).

Please note that the prevalence of trisomy 21 at this state of pregnancy is almost twice as high as the prevalence in livebirths, because 40-45% of pregnancies with affected fetuses result in spontaneous miscarriage.

1. What is the screening test shown in the report? What is the purpose of using it? At what gestational age would you organise it? (3 marks)

2.   What is the normal value of this screening test? (1 mark)

3.   Name three conditions you might associate with abnormal result. (3 marks)

4.   What is the indication for this test in this case? (1 mark)

5.   Name two methods which can be used to confirm the diagnosis. (2 marks)

11

You are the hospital doctor and you receive the following letter:

> *The Surgery*
> *2 The Street*
> *Anywhere*
>
> *Dear Doctor*
>
> **Re: Mrs A. J. aged 28**
>
> *June has been happily married for the last five years, and intercourse had caused no problems. Recently she has developed marked discomfort with intercourse.*
>
> *I would be grateful for your expert opinion.*
>
> *Yours sincerely*
>
> *Dr A Jones*

1. List four questions which may help you to make a diagnosis.
    (4 marks)

2. List three abnormalities you may find on examination that will help you make the diagnosis. (3 marks)

3. List two investigations you may perform. (2 marks)

4. Which other health professional would be useful to the woman? (1 mark)

12

Look at the illustration.

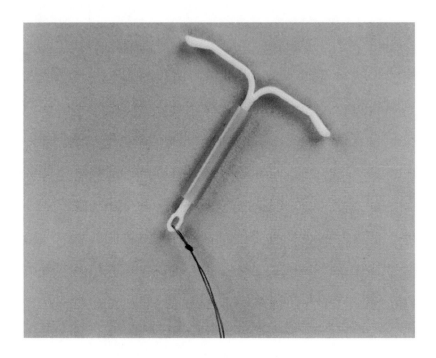

1.   What hormone is released by the above coil? (1 mark)

2.   What is the reliability of this coil? (1 mark)

3. How long will it work for? (1 mark)

4. What may happen to the woman's periods with this coil *in situ*? (1 mark)

5. You examine the woman for a smear six months post-insertion and the strings are lost. What two investigations may be helpful? (2 marks)

6. If you find she is eight weeks pregnant what will you do with the coil if the strings cannot be seen? (1 mark)

7. What are the potential risks of this pregnancy? (2 marks)

8.   What is the risk of an ectopic pregnancy? (1 mark)

13

Look at Mrs B. J.'s partogram.

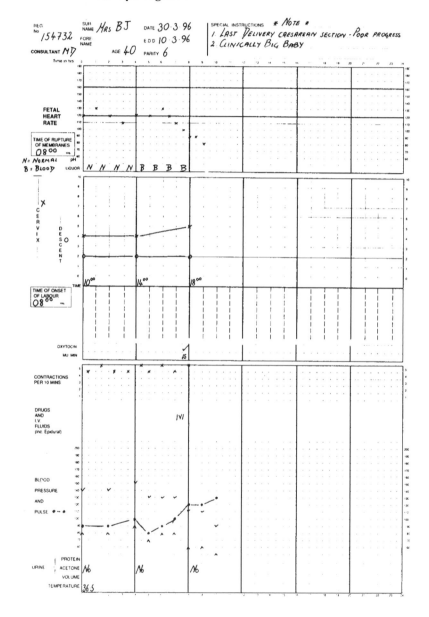

1. What would concern you before Mrs B. J. went into labour?
    (2 marks)

2. What would be the best management at 1400 hrs? (1 mark)

3. What was done wrong at 1800 hrs? (1 mark)

4. What is the most probable diagnosis of what happens after 1800 hrs?
    (1 mark)

5. How could this have been avoided? (1 mark)

6. Give two methods of assessing intrapartum fetal wellbeing. (2 marks)

7. What advice would you give to Mrs B. J. with regards to future pregnancy? (2 marks)

14

You are a hospital doctor who receives the following:

```
DEPARTMENT OF HISTOPATHOLOGY & CYTOLOGY

NAME         :                          PATIENT ID NO :
PREVIOUS NAME :                         LAB NO        :
DOB          : 15/NOV/1982             GP CODE       :

CONSULTANT/GP :             Cons Obs
??           : COLPOSCOPY
COPY TO      :                          GROV
-------------------------------------------------------------------------
Specimen Date   : 05/Dec/2002           Received Date : 05/Dec/2002

Specimen(s)     : CERVICAL SMEAR

Clinical Details : ON O/C. PREV BORDERLINE. TODAY BX

Cytology Report : MODERATELY DYSKARYOTIC CELLS SUGGESTIVE OF CIN II
                  PERSIST. **ACTION REQUIRED**

                : 3S

Report Date     : 19/Dec/2002
```

1. What would you do next? (1 mark)

2. Who is eligible for cervical screening? How often should women have a smear? (2 marks)

3. How can a diagnosis be made? (1 mark)

4. Give two methods for the treatment of CIN. (2 marks)

5. List four risk factors for cervical cancer. (4 marks)

15

You are a hospital doctor and you receive the following letter:

> Dr J Smith
> The Old Manor Medical Centre
> The Street
> Little Somewhere
> Crumbleshire
> JS/abc
>
> 3 December 1995
>
> Dear Richard
>
> **Re: Mrs T. L., d.o.b. 30.3.57**
>
> Many thanks indeed for seeing this very pleasant air hostess who spends a lot of time crossing the Atlantic.
>
> Her husband, Michael, I believe you were at school with and is a regular golfing partner of yours.
>
> She has recently undergone a third attempt at IVF, the last two failed, and I am delighted to say that she is now pregnant.
>
> LMP was 19 August 1995 and this is her first pregnancy.
>
> She is very keen to be under your care and knows that you are away on holiday for the next three weeks, but is happy to wait to see you on your return.
>
> All best wishes
> Yours sincerely
>
>
> Dr J. Smith
>
>
> PS Apart from the insulin for her diabetes, she is well.

1. List four clinical things that concern you about this pregnancy. (4 marks)

2. How has the referring doctor mis-managed this patient? (1 mark)

3. Give three specific congenital abnormalities or findings you are looking for in Mrs T. L.'s case when you ask for an ultrasound scan at 19 weeks. (3 marks)

4. How would you plan the rest of Mrs T. L.'s care? (2 marks)

16

Miss T. H. is a 32-year-old P2+1. Her LMP was 4–5 weeks ago. She presents to your clinic with mild vaginal bleeding for two days and a positive urinary pregnancy test. Her transabdominal scan report (she declined transvaginal scan) shows:

> *Anteverted uterus containing a single intrauterine gestation sac of mean diameter 11 mm (5–6 week size).*
> *No fetal pole seen as yet. Normal ovaries. No free fluid.*
> *No obvious cause for p.v. bleed seen.*
> *A further scan is suggested in 2 weeks to reassess viability.*
>
> *Reviewed and electronically signed by*
> *Senior Radiographer*

Miss T. H. is very tearful and anxious about this pregnancy. She has a list of questions for you:

1. Miss T. H. asks you if she is still pregnant. What is your answer? (2 marks)

2. Miss T. H. wondered what she can do to stop her bleeding. What is your answer? (2 marks)

3. Miss T. H. is anxious and would like you to tell her about her chance of having a miscarriage if she is still pregnant. If she is still pregnant, what do you say? (2 marks)

4. Miss T. H. asks you about the causes of miscarriages. List three common causes. (3 marks)

5. How would you manage Miss T. H.'s condition? (1 mark)

17

This photograph shows a set of instruments commonly used in labour ward

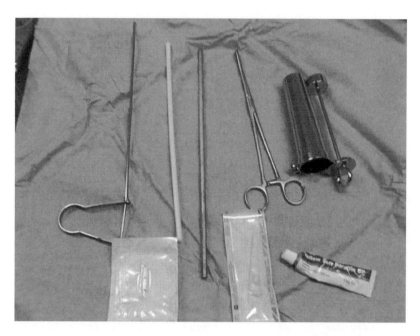

1. What is this set used for? (1 mark)

2. Name two abnormalities in the cardiotocograph which indicate the use of these instruments? (2 marks)

3. List three contraindications for this procedure. (3 marks)

| |
| |
| |
| |

4. List two possible complications for this procedure. (2 marks)

| |
| |
| |

5. Regarding the result of this procedure. What is the normal value? What type of value would you act on? (2 marks)

| |
| |
| |

18

You have been asked to discuss pain relief in labour with a couple. They are keen to be fully informed.

1. List two non-pharmacological methods of pain relief. (2 marks)

2. List three other methods of pain relief and beside each one list a contraindication or side-effect. (6 marks)

Method of pain relief	Contraindication/ side-effect
1.	1.
2.	2.
3.	3.

3. What syndrome is associated with aspiration of gastric contents? (1 mark)

4. How can this be avoided? (1 mark)

19

Mrs S. D. is a 75-year-old lady who presented to your clinic with a history of urinary incontinence for the past three years. Her symptoms have worsened recently and she says that she hardly goes out. She has been on hormone replacement therapy for more than 10 years. She had a vaginal hysterectomy in 1985 with repair and also had an anterior colporrhaphy in 1987. She had an appendicectomy in 1988.

1. List three questions you would ask Mrs S. D. following the above history to identify the cause of her incontinence? (3 marks)

Genuine stress incontinence is the most common cause of urinary incontinence in women.

2. Give three indications for conservative treatment. (3 marks)

3. Name two conservative treatment methods can be used for stress incontinence. (2 marks)

An overactive bladder, the second most common cause of urinary incontinence in women, affects 30% of incontinent women.

4. Name two methods for the treatment of detrusor instability. (2 marks)

20

Look at the photograph below.

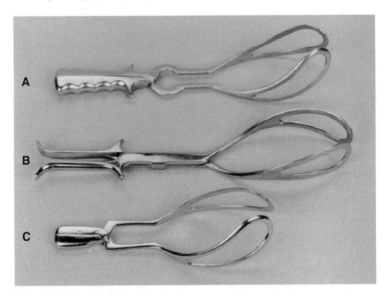

1.   Name the three forceps shown in the picture. (3 marks)

2. List four requirements that must be satisfied before a forceps delivery. (4 marks)

3.   What is shown in the photograph below? (1 mark)

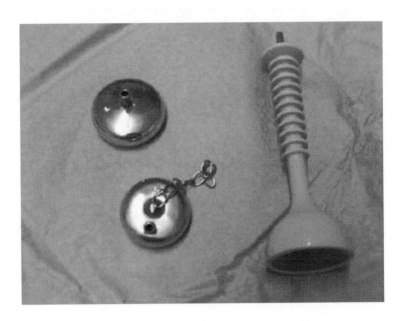

4.   Give two advantages of the use of this instrument against the use of forceps. (2 marks)

OSCE Practice Exam 2:
Answers and Teaching Notes

1

Antepartum haemorrhage is bleeding from the genital tract after 24 weeks' gestation. *The Confidential Enquiry into Maternal Death in the UK 1997–1999* reveals haemorrhage to be a significant cause of direct maternal death. The incidence is 3% of all pregnancies: approximately 1% due to placenta previa, 1% due to abruptio placentae and 1% due to other causes. Other causes include cervical ectropion, cervical polyps, cervical cancer, vulval varicosities and uterine rupture.

Transvaginal ultrasound (TVS) is safe in the presence of placenta praevia and is more accurate than transabdominal ultrasound (TAS) in locating the placenta. In the second trimester transabdominal ultrasound is associated with very high numbers of false-positive diagnoses for placenta praevia and although third-trimester scans can improve on this, they are still associated with significant errors. Transvaginal sonography can improve on this diagnosis.

Women who have had a Caesarean section in a previous pregnancy and who have a placenta praevia subsequently should be considered at high risk of having a morbidly adherent placenta (placenta accreta) or ruptured uterus.

Management includes:

a.   Blood transfusion. Prior to delivery all women with placenta praevia and their partners should have had discussions regarding delivery and possible blood transfusion requirements and any objections or queries should have been dealt with effectively.

b.   Possibility of hysterectomy.

Senior anaesthetic, obstetric and paediatric input are vital in planning the delivery. When a woman with placenta praevia is being delivered, the consultant on-call for the delivery suite should be involved.

2

These cases represent the different types of dysmenorrhoea (ie painful menstruation). Secondary dysmenorrhoea, which occurs with Mrs P. T., occurs in older women and results from underlying pelvic pathology. Endometriosis, chronic pelvic inflammatory disease, fibroids, or occasionally the presence of an intrauterine contraceptive device, can be the underlying pathology.

Investigations can be difficult. An ultrasound scan can be useful for helping to diagnose fibroids, but eventually a diagnostic laparoscopy may be useful in differentiating between endometriosis and pelvic inflammatory disease. Hopefully, the presence of a coil would have been presented in the history.

The different medical treatments obviously depend on the pathology that is detected. Endometriosis can be treated hormonally by the following:

- continuous combined oral contraceptive pill

- progestogens

- danazol

- gestrinone

- luteinising hormone releasing hormone analogues.

Chronic pelvic inflammatory disease is difficult to treat medically, as are fibroids.

Hannah, her 15-year-old daughter, has primary dysmenorrhoea. This occurs in young women with the onset of ovulation and without any specific underlying pathology. It appears that biochemical changes that occur in the menstrual cycle initiate some form of uterine ischaemia due to vasospasm and the pain is secondary to myometrial contractions. In the box you could write 'ovulation', or 'biochemical changes associated with the menstrual cycle'.

Primary dysmenorrhoea can be treated by either the use of the combined oral contraceptive pill to prevent ovulation or with mefenamic acid in high doses (500 mg, three times a day) ideally to start a couple of days before the onset of the pain. Mefenamic acid is a prostaglandin synthesase inhibitor and if this is ineffective, other inhibitors can be tried.

3

The main problem with Joanna is that she has not had a period for five months. We are, therefore, looking at possible causes of amenorrhoea. Physiological causes of amenorrhoea include pregnancy and the menopause. It is, therefore, important to do a pregnancy test and to check her follicle-stimulating hormone (FSH), luteinising hormone (LH) levels and serum oestradiol.

Important questions to ask her include:

- When did her periods start?

- Are they always irregular or is this a new problem?

- Does she have any postcoital or intermenstrual bleeding?

- Does she have tender breasts?

- Does she have any milk coming from her breasts?

- Does she suffer from hot flushes or night sweats?

- Has she experienced any nausea or vomiting?

- Has she noticed any changes to her eyesight?

- Has she lost her sense of smell?

- Has there been any change in her weight?

- Has she noticed any excessive hair growth or spots?

- What drugs is she on?

Hormonal problems include hyperprolactinaemia, which will be detected by an elevated prolactin, and hypogonadotrophic hypogonadism (eg Kallman's syndrome). This would also be detected by a low FSH and LH, with a low oestradiol but may require more dynamic testing.

Polycystic ovarian syndrome, weight loss, chronic illness and psychogenic causes are also possible. Many of the drugs used in psychiatry raise prolactin levels. Hypothyroidism can lead to amenorrhoea and may also be associated with elevated prolactin levels. Asherman's syndrome may develop following a miscarriage and especially after an evacuation for retained products of conception.

The blood tests indicate hyperprolactinaemia and the important test to do at this stage is computed tomography of the pituitary fossa to look for micro- and macroadenomas. Some units take an X-ray of the pituitary fossa, whereas others perform magnetic resonance imaging.

Joanna can have medical or surgical treatment. Hyperprolactinaemia can be treated surgically, although this is rarely done. Dopamine agonists (eg bromocriptine or cabergoline) have now become the primary modality used to treat micro- and macroadenomas of the pituitary. Bromocriptine (an ergot derivative) acts by decreasing the secretion and synthesis of prolactin by the lactotrophs and also causes a reduction in the cytoplasmic volume of the lactotrophs.

The side-effects of bromocriptine can be severe and these include gastrointestinal symptoms, such as nausea and vomiting, and cardiovascular effects, such as dizziness and syncope. Less common complications include headache, nasal congestion, abdominal cramps and constipation. In very high doses, confusion, hallucinations and even seizures have been reported. Once weekly cabergoline may produce fewer side-effects.

There is much controversy about what is the best form of treatment for a woman who falls pregnant whilst on bromocriptine. There appears to be no evidence that bromocriptine is teratogenic or that there is an increased fetal loss; however, therapy generally should be discontinued during pregnancy.

Only 1% of microadenomas progress during pregnancy, but macroadenomas have a greater risk of expanding. Patients with macroadenomas need to be carefully monitored and treatment should be reinitiated if symptoms such as headache or visual-field disturbance occur.

4

This is obviously a case of severe pre-eclampsia. This is associated with cerebral haemorrhage and is a major cause of maternal death.

There are several things you should do. An examination is required to assess the clonus and hyper-reflexia and other signs of pre-eclamptic toxaemia.

It is essential that this patient be admitted to hospital via an ambulance as a matter of urgency and a telephone call to the hospital should be made. It may be advisable for an antihypertensive treatment to be given before transfer.

At the hospital it would be important to stabilise the blood pressure, monitor the wellbeing of the baby and assess the mother's wellbeing, including assessing renal function by monitoring the urinary output and urea, electrolytes and urate. Liver function needs to be assessed by liver function tests. Hydralazine and magnesium sulphate are useful for acute reduction of blood pressure as is nifedipine, which can be given sublingually. Magnesium sulphate may reduce the incidence of eclampsia. All are associated with a headache. Blood pressure control can be maintained using either labetalol or methyldopa. The risk of disseminated intravascular coagulation needs to be assessed and this includes bloods for platelets and a full clotting screen.

From the above, answers to the question 'What will you do' include:

- Full examination of patient
- Arrange admission to hospital via ambulance
- Contact 'on call team' at hospital re transfer to hospital
- Consider control of blood pressure.

Tests and actions which should be performed in hospital include:

- Cardiotocography
- Doppler blood flow
- Ultrasound to assess fetal growth and well-being via a biophysical profile
- Stabilise blood pressure
- Review anticonvulsant therapy
- Assess liver function

- Assess renal function
- Assess evidence of disseminated intravascular coagulation.

In order to decide the best route of delivery, a vaginal examination should be performed to see if the woman is favourable for induction.

Before any form of delivery it is important to do a clotting screen. This is especially important if one needs to do a Caesarean section or if an epidural, which is the preferred method of pain relief, is given.

Once the patient is delivered she is still at risk from an eclamptic fit for up to 48 hours. The clotting factors, urinary output and blood pressure must be watched carefully and careful fluid management is important because the patient may become polyuric with haemoconcentration. A central venous line is advisable.

Good answers to the question of postpartum monitoring include:

- Monitor blood pressure
- Monitor urinary output
- Monitor fluid balance
- Monitor clotting screens.

5

An episode of bleeding 12 months or more after the last period is accepted as postmenopausal bleeding. (Also some authors will accept that any vaginal bleeding six months or more after the last period is accepted as postmenopausal bleeding).

Gynaecological malignancies must be ruled out in any case of post-menopausal bleeding. Endometrial cancer is present in approximately 5–10% of patients with postmenopausal bleeding. It must be remembered that postmenopausal bleeding may also be the presenting symptom of cervical cancer and some ovarian cancers. The most common benign disorders causing postmenopausal bleeding are hormone replacement therapy, atrophic vaginitis, atrophic endometrium, endometrial polyps, endometrial hyperplasia and cervical lesions.

Transvaginal ultrasound has been used to detect endometrial carcinoma by measuring the thickness of the endometrium. In general, a negative transvaginal ultrasound result (endometrial thickness of 5 mm or less) reduces the risk of significant disease (endometrial cancer) by 84%. Endometrial cancer is the most common gynaecological malignancy and the fourth most common malignancy in women after breast, colorectal and lung cancer.

The aetiology of endometrial cancer is unknown, but several factors are known to increase the risk of developing endometrial cancer. The median age of patient with endometrial cancer is 60 years, with 80% being post-menopausal and only 3–5% being less than 40 years old. Women with endometrial cancer are often obese, nulliparous, with diabetes or hyper-tension and history of early menarche or late menopause. Unopposed oestrogen replacement will increase the relative risk of endometrial carcinoma by around six-fold after five years of use. Women receiving tamoxifen in the treatment or prevention of breast cancer experience a three- to six-fold greater incidence of endometrial cancer. Women with hereditary non-polyposis colorectal cancer (HNPCC) are at risk of devel-oping endometrial cancer. The estimated lifetime risk of developing endometrial cancer in women carrying these mutations is around 42–60%.

Formerly, the principal means of hospital investigation was by dilatation and curettage (D&C), but newer methods of investigation such as out-patient endometrial biopsy and out-patient hysteroscopy have superseded D&C. Endometrial biopsy can be undertaken using endometrial samplers (pipelle, Z-sampler). Out-patient endometrial sampling has a procedure failure rate as well as a tissue-yield failure rate, each of approximately 10%. Hysteroscopy in the out-patient setting appears to have an accuracy and patient acceptability equivalent to in-patient hysteroscopy under general anaesthetic. Hysteroscopy is the current gold standard and the preferred diagnostic technique to detect polyps and other benign lesions. The need to perform a cervical smear should never be forgotten.

6

In the UK approximately 30% of all couples choose sterilisation as a method of contraception, rising to almost 50% of those aged over 40. Despite being a very common procedure, sterilisation is still considered a major area of litigation and medico-legal complaint. The following consent issues should be covered in detail:

- Alternative long-term contraceptive methods should be discussed in detail. This includes failure rates, advantages and disadvantages of each method.

- Women seeking sterilisation should be advised that the procedure is intended to be permanent.

- Failure rate or risk of pregnancy following the procedure should be mentioned. This is approximately 1:200 in her lifetime and pregnancy can occur several years after the procedure. If the procedure failed, there is a high risk of ectopic pregnancy.

- Risks of laparoscopy (such as bowel and bladder injury) and the chances of requiring laparotomy.

- Women must be advised to continue to use effective contraception until their next (post-procedure) period.

Although there are procedures to reverse female sterilisation, the operation is complex and expensive and the success rate depends on several factors (such as the surgeon's experience with the reversal procedure, age of the client, the type of sterilisation the client received, average tubal length, and site of anastomosis).

Although some studies have reported high success rates, the live birth rates are lower than the 'success' rates reported.

A study looking at sterilisation reversals in women over 40 found a live birth rate of 14.3% and a spontaneous abortion rate of 23.8%.

Tubal occlusion is not associated with an increased risk of heavier or irregular periods. Women must be advised to continue to use effective contraception until their next (post-procedure) period.

Follow up at her GP surgery 5–7 days following sterilisation is strongly recommended to check on the healing of the wound and to remove any sutures. The woman should be advised to come back if she has any problems (fever, pain, bleeding and discharge) or at any time if she has questions or concerns.

7

This is an ultrasound fetal growth chart or fetal growth chart.

There are two main components: head circumference (above) and abdominal circumference (below).

Asymmetrical intrauterine growth retardation is seen. In this situation the head circumference is relatively spared.

Methods employed to detect small for gestational age fetuses include abdominal palpation, measurement of symphyseal fundal height, ultrasound biometry, ultrasound estimated fetal weight and ultrasound Doppler flow velocimetry.

Maternal causes include:

- Chronic illness: any debilitating disease in the mother increases the risk of having asymmetrical growth retardation. This may be because of deprivation of nutrients or oxygen available to the placenta. As medical care improves many women with disease (eg cystic fibrosis, congenital heart disease, or renal failure after transplant) are now presenting in pregnancy.

- Smoking in pregnancy

- Alcohol

- Illegal drugs

- Haemoglobinopathies, such as sickle cell disease

- Collagen vascular disease, such as systemic lupus erythematosus.

Fetuses are at greater risk of stillbirth, birth hypoxia, neonatal complications, impaired neurodevelopment and possibly type 2 (non-insulin-dependent) diabetes and hypertension in adult life.

8

Serum α-fetoprotein testing (AFP) is available at 16 weeks and, if elevated, is a screening test for open neural tube defects. The diagnostic test is by a detailed ultrasound scan in the second trimester.

True incidence of congenital malformations of the heart is uncertain, but probably lies between 5 and 8 per 1000 births. Up to 60% of these can be detected by an ultrasound scan, but a significant number are not detected until early infancy.

One can be suspicious of congenital heart disease in the newborn if the baby presents in one of the following ways:

- Cardiac failure with tachypnoea, costal recession, tachycardia, peripheral oedema and enlargement of the liver

- Cyanosis

- A cardiac murmur

- An arrhythmia

- General failure to thrive.

The instance of congenital dislocation of the hip is in the order of 1–2 per 1000 births.

Congenital dislocation of the hip is more likely in girls than in boys and is more likely in babies born with a breech presentation. The incidence also increases if there is a family history of this condition.

Phenylketonuria occurs once per 10 000–15 000 births, but once identified, early treatment can prevent mental handicap.

9

The differential diagnosis is placenta praevia or placental abruption. Abruption is the diagnosis in this case. (Placenta praevia is excluded by an ultrasound scan.)

Placental abruption can be life-threatening to both baby and mother and it is important to act quickly. The most important actions that should be taken include putting a drip up and sending blood off for investigations. The investigations should include a full blood count, checking for a coagulation defect and cross-matching up to six units of blood.

Another important action is to check the well-being of the fetus and this would include cardiotocography. Obviously, checking the wellbeing of the mother should include blood pressure, pulse and urinary output. Any of these points would be appropriate answers to Question 2.

If the pain and bleeding increase this demonstrates that the placental abruption is persisting and one is always concerned about the development of disseminated intravascular coagulation (DIC) from which maternal death usually ensues.

Delivery is usually by Caesarean section, but before this a vaginal examination should be carried out in case a vaginal delivery may be performed. This must *not* be done until placenta praevia has been excluded by ultrasound scan. It is essential to exclude DIC prior to any surgery.

Patients who have had an antepartum haemorrhage are more likely to develop postpartum bleeding.

Good answers to Question 3 would be:

- Consider delivery
- Stabilise mother
- Assess wellbeing of baby
- Check for DIC.

Syntocinon may be useful in these cases. Remember that the ergometrine may be associated with a rise in blood pressure and should not be given in patients who are pre-eclamptic.

Carboprost is useful in postpartum haemorrhage due to uterine relaxation and is useful in patients who are unresponsive to ergometrine and oxytocin. Great caution should be used in patients who are hypertensive.

If the bleeding continues despite medical treatment then very careful monitoring of the coagulation products should be performed. Also, consider examination of the patient under anaesthetic, assessment for retained products of conception and, eventually, a postpartum hysterectomy.

10

Nuchal translucency (NT) is a term used to describe a sonolucent area in the nuchal region (back of the neck) of the fetus and is typically observed in the first trimester. Nuchal translucency screening provides a couple with an individual specific risk for having a child with Down's syndrome, trisomy 13 and trisomy 18. To obtain risk assessment using NT and age, it is critical that the NT be measured between 11 weeks, 0 days and 13 weeks, 6 days.

Increased NT refers to a NT measurement of > 3 mm. This does not mean that the fetus has a chromosome abnormality. But it does mean that the fetus is at an increased risk for some disorders and birth defects.

Increased NT thickness is associated with:

a.   Chromosome aneuploidy, including trisomies 21 (Down's syndrome), 18, 13 and triploidy and Turner's syndrome (45 XO)

b.   Among karyotypically normal fetuses with NT > 3 mm, there is a greater risk for birth defects, including cardiovascular (cardiac septal defects) and pulmonary defects (diaphragmatic hernia), renal defects and abdominal wall defects (eg omphalocele).

c.   Other causes of increased NT:

- Noonan's syndrome
- Smith–Lemli–Opitz syndrome
- Stickler's syndrome
- Jarcho–Levine syndrome
- Miller–Dieker syndrome.

Increased maternal age is the indication in this case. The association between Down's syndrome and increased maternal age was noticed in 1909 by Shuttleworth.

Three variables are taken into consideration for determining a woman's risk for having a child with a chromosomal abnormality.

Maternal age: The risk for a fetal chromosomal abnormality increases with increasing maternal age.

Gestational age: The risk for fetal chromosomal abnormalities decreases with increasing gestational age.

Previous fetus or baby with trisomy: The risk for fetal chromosomal abnormalities increases the age-related risk by 0.75% or 1 in 150.

The following issues should be considered during interpretation of the result:

- The nuchal translucency test is only a screening test that aims to give a risk of a particular woman having a chromosomal disorder.

- A low risk cannot exclude Down's syndrome or other chromosomal disorders.

- The test will pick up 80% of pregnancies affected by Down's syndrome.

- The test itself does not carry any risk to the mother or the baby.

- If a test is positive (ie recalculated risk is greater than 1:300) an invasive test is usually recommended to determine the baby's chromosomal pattern.

11

Dyspareunia is a very common problem that presents not only to the gynaecologist, but also to the general practitioner. Questioning should be directed towards finding out initially whether the pain is superficial, ie pain on penetration or deeper. You need to ask when the pain is occurring and if it is in a particular position.

Superficial dyspareunia may be due to an anatomical problem within the vulva, vagina, or urethra, or may be more psychosexual in origin. Deep dyspareunia is associated with ovarian cysts, chronic or acute pelvic inflammatory disease, ectopic pregnancies, or endometriosis.

It would, therefore, be useful to ask questions on vaginal discharge and bleeding. In this case anatomical causes are unlikely as Mrs A. J. has, in the past, had intercourse without any problems. The development of a Bartholin's abscess, cyst, or vulval lichen sclerosis may be associated with the problems.

The history of her periods would be important because this may be associated with endometriosis. Pelvic inflammatory disease is associated with lower abdominal pain and a vaginal discharge.

Appropriate answers to Question 1 include:

- Is the pain on entrance or deep penetration?
- What are your periods like?
- Is there any position that makes it worse?
- Any abnormal swelling?
- Any discharge?
- When was your last period?
- Any vaginal swelling?
- Any vulval itching?

Questioning needs to be done very sympathetically and several consultations may be required before one feels that the answer has been obtained.

The examination may reveal no abnormality at all or may demonstrate a vaginal discharge associated with an infection or even atrophic vaginitis if there is the association with premature menopause.

A pelvic mass such as a fibroid or an ovarian cyst may also be found on pelvic examination.

Endometriosis can be detected by a tender uterus and utero-sacral thickening and pelvic inflammatory disease may also be suspected if examination reveals lower abdominal discomfort and a vaginal discharge.

Investigations that can be helpful include an ultrasound scan, although this is not always as useful as one would hope initially, but a laparoscopy in cases of deep dyspareunia is very useful. If there is an indication that there may be an infective origin then high vaginal, endocervical and urethral swabs would be helpful.

It is important at an early stage to get the help of a psychosexual counsellor because even if an anatomical cause is detected there may be some psychosexual element to the problem and the problem itself could actually cause a psychosexual problem.

12

The picture shows the hormonal intrauterine system (IUS) which is an effective, long-term and reversible method of contraception. It consists of a small plastic T-shaped frame which is inserted into the womb. This carries the hormone levonorgestrel in a sleeve around its stem and has two fine threads attached to the base. The hormone is gradually released into the uterus and the rate of release is controlled by the special covering on the hormone sleeve.

Levonorgestrel works by keeping the lining of the womb thin, and thickening the cervical mucus to prevent sperm penetration. In some women, ovulation is also prevented.

The IUS is a very reliable method of contraception. Studies have shown that if 1000 women use this system for one year, no more than two may become pregnant. This is very similar to sterilisation.

The system is effective for five years and its reliability remains the same throughout the five years. In the UK it is now licensed for five years.

The IUS will affect the woman's periods. Many women will have spotting or light vaginal bleeding in addition to their periods for the first 3–6 months after the system is fitted. Some women may have heavy or prolonged bleeding during this time. Overall, there is gradually a reduction in the number of bleeding days and the amount of blood lost each month. Some women eventually find that their periods stop altogether. This amenorrhoea is not a cause for concern as the circulating oestradiol levels are not affected and, therefore, osteoporosis does not occur. One mark is available for your answer to Question 4, and an answer such as 'Gradual reduction and possibly amenorrhea occurs in most women' would be sufficient.

If the coil strings are not found then there is a concern that either the strings are lost or the coil has fallen out. The major causes of lost strings include perforation and a pregnancy. It is useful to have a urinary pregnancy test, an ultrasound scan and an X-ray of the pelvis.

Your answer to Question 6 could be 'Nothing' or 'Do not try to remove the coil and monitor the pregnancy carefully'.

In the above case, as the coil strings are lost there is nothing one can do about the woman being pregnant. She does run the risk of second-trimester abortion and premature labour. If the strings are visualised and she is still in the first 12 weeks then removal should be considered.

Although this creates a risk of miscarriage, this risk is less than if you leave the coil *in situ*.

It does appear that with the levonorgestrel coil the risk of ectopic pregnancies is decreased.

13

This is a case of uterine rupture.

The important features about this partogram are that Mrs B. J. had a previous Caesarean section due to failure to progress at 5 cm and is known to have a large baby this time. She is also a grandmultipara (six previous children), aged 40. Obviously the management of her labour should have been discussed before the commencement of labour. She is also 20 days past her dates.

To summarise, your answer to the first part of this question about your concerns should include two of the following:

- Large baby
- Previous Caesarean section
- Grand multiparity
- Post dates
- Her age

At 1400 h a Caesarean section would have been the preferred management. However, if it was decided that a trial of scar was to be performed then it would have been important to have put in an intravenous cannula and 'grouped and saved' the patient. This should have been done on admission.

At 1800 h it was totally inappropriate to put up oxytocin, because of the evidence of uterine rupture and also because the patient is a grand multip.

After good contractions Mrs B. J. had only dilated 1 cm and there was no descent of the head. Most traumatic ruptures of the uterus are associated with inappropriate oxytocin use. After 1830 h it becomes quite evident, with a falling fetal heart, a maternal tachycardia and hypotension, that uterine rupture is occurring and the presence of blood within the liquor is an important diagnostic pointer.

This traumatic event could have been avoided by performing an elective Caesarean section. This is the answer to Question 5.

Routine methods of assessing intrapartum fetal wellbeing include intermittent fetal auscultation, cardiotocography and, if necessary, fetal scalp pH monitoring.

In Mrs B. J.'s case, immediate delivery of this baby would be by an emergency Caesarean section.

She has now had two Caesarean sections and one uterine rupture. Obviously advice concerning future pregnancies depends on the extent of the uterine rupture. It may well be advisable for her not to get pregnant again, but if she insisted on getting pregnant then careful monitoring and an elective Caesarean section at around 37 weeks is possibly indicated.

Also, note her age risks need to be discussed. Your answer to the question about the advice you give to Mrs B. J. with regards to future pregnancy should include any two of the following:

- Counselling about the dangers of rupture of the uterus, including recurrence.

- Need for elective Caesarean section.

- Age-related risks with future pregnancy.

- You may consider advising her to avoid another pregnancy.

14

This patient needs to be referred to the colposcopy clinic for colposcopic examination and cervical biopsy.

All women between the ages of 20 and 64 are eligible for a free cervical smear test every 3–5 years. Around 60% of health authorities invite women every three years and 15% have a mixed policy, inviting women every 3 or 5 years, depending upon their age.

Cervical screening began in Britain in the mid-1960s. By the mid-1980s, although many women were having regular smear tests, there was concern that those at greatest risk were not being tested, and that those who had positive results were not being followed up and treated effectively. The NHS Cervical Screening Programme was set up in 1988 when the Department of Health instructed all health authorities to introduce computerised call–recall systems and to meet certain quality standards.

The diagnosis can be confirmed by taking a colposcopy directed biopsy for the histological examination.

The programme screens almost 4 million women in England each year. Of the 3.6 million screened in 2000–2001, 2.4 million were tested following an invitation and 1.2 million were screened. There were 2740 new cases of invasive cervical cancer in England and Wales in 1997. This is a 26% fall in incidence over the previous five years with 9.3 cases per 100 000 women. According to the Imperial Cancer Research Fund, cervical screening prevents between 1100 and 3900 cases of cervical cancer each year. The UK has the second highest recorded incidence in the European community.

The following can be used to treat CIN:

- Large loop excision of the transformation zone.

- Laser

- Cold coagulation

- Knife cone biopsy.

Diathermy and cryocautery are not recommended.

Cervical cancer is the 12th most common cause of cancer deaths in women in the UK. The exact cause of cervical cancer is not known. However, it is known that:

- Certain types of human papillomavirus are linked with around 95% of all cases of cervical cancer.

- Women with many sexual partners or whose partners have had many partners, are more at risk.

- Using a condom gives some protection; long-term use of the pill may increase the risk.

- Women who smoke are about twice as likely to develop the disease as non-smokers.

- Women with a late first pregnancy have a lower risk than those with an early pregnancy; the risk rises with the number of pregnancies.

- Women in manual social classes are at higher risk that those in non-manual social classes.

15

This very pleasant referral letter totally misses the point and, therefore, is putting the patient's care at risk.

She has been referred late, and is now over 15 weeks into what must be classed as a high-risk pregnancy. Also, she is an insulin-dependent diabetic and this is only documented as an afterthought in the referring letter which is more concerned with pleasantries than with medical fact.

There are several things that would be of concern about this patient. These include:

- She is 38 years of age and obviously at greater risk of Down's syndrome.

- She is spending a lot of time crossing the Atlantic and, therefore, needs some counselling about her job.

- She has an *in vitro* fertilisation pregnancy and is at risk of multiple pregnancy which is important if she is considering flying.

- She is a diabetic and needs to be seen early to optimise blood glucose control and be linked up with a joint obstetric/diabetic clinic.

This patient should have been referred much earlier.

On ultrasound scanning the congenital abnormalities associated with pregnancy may be detected and these include sacral agenesis and cardiac abnormalities. Markers for Down's syndrome could also be detected, which include congenital heart defects as well as increased nuchal fold thickness. Multiple pregnancy should also be looked for.

The management of Mrs T. L.'s case obviously depends on whether she has a single or multiple pregnancy.

Early booking would be advisable including hospital care at the joint obstetric/diabetic clinic. The aim is to optimise blood glucose levels. Serial scans for growth need to be performed, as well as monitoring for polyhydramnios which may be an indication of poor diabetic control.

She is also at risk of pre-eclampsia and close monitoring of this is important. Consider not allowing the pregnancy to proceed past 38–40 weeks.

Good answers to Question 4 include:

- Book into a joint obstetric/diabetic clinic
- Detailed booking ultrasound scan
- Regular ultrasound scans for growth
- Increase surveillance for pre-eclampsia
- Regular HbA1C measurement
- Have paediatrician in attendance at delivery.

16

It is difficult to answer this question with a definite yes or no. Miss T. H. has a positive pregnancy test and her pelvic scan show an early gestational sac which may present as a normal healthy pregnancy. However, her mild bleeding may indicate an early sign of disruption of ongoing pregnancy. In the presence of her mild bleeding and absence of any significant abdominal pain, repeat scan in two weeks to confirm location and viability of this pregnancy.

Sadly, there is little that can be done to stop a miscarriage progressing. Clinical management has changed little in the last five decades and has commonly been based on tradition rather than a sound evidence-base. An example of this was the use of bed-rest, which does not affect the outcome in threatened miscarriage.

It is possible that as many as 50% of pregnancies miscarry before implantation. Miscarriage is known to occur in 10–20% of clinical pregnancies and accounts for 50 000 in-patient admissions to hospital in the United Kingdom annually.

Earlier miscarriage is most likely caused by chromosomal abnormality including trisomy, polyploidy and autosomal monosomy. This accounts for 60% of spontaneous miscarriages during the first eight weeks. Other factors which contribute to early miscarriage are:

- Acute maternal illness, eg pyrexia.

- Infections, eg toxoplasmosis, other infections, rubella, cytomegalovirus infection and herpes simplex (TORCH)

- Chronic maternal diseases (hypertension, thyroid dysfunction systemic lupus erythematosus and diabetes).

- Smoking and alcohol.

Reassure her and organise another scan in 10 days to confirm location and viability of this pregnancy. Also advise her to attend the hospital if her bleeding or pain increase.

17

This is a fetal blood sample set. Other names include fetal scalp blood and scalp pH testing. This is a transvaginal procedure performed during active labour, where the fetal scalp is cleaned and a small fetal blood sample is taken for pH evaluation. The procedure typically takes about five minutes.

Where delivery is contemplated because of an abnormal fetal heart rate pattern, or in cases of suspected fetal acidosis, fetal blood sampling should be undertaken. These may include complicated fetal tachycardia, fetal bradycardia, persistent late decelerations, loss of variability and persistent variable decelerations.

Contraindications to fetal blood sampling include:

- Maternal infection (eg human immunodeficiency virus, hepatitis viruses and herpes simplex virus) in these cases, the procedure increases the risk of transmitting infection to the fetus.

- Fetal bleeding disorders

- Prematurity (< 34 weeks).

Risks include infection, fetal scalp bruising and, in very rare circumstances, continuous bleeding from fetal scalp.

The normal fetal blood pH is between 7.25 and 7.35. If the fetal blood pH is between 7.20 and 7.25 the recommendation is to repeat fetal blood sample within 30 minutes or consider delivery if there has been a rapid fall since the last sample. Value < 7.20 indicates urgent delivery.

18

There is a wide range of methods available to give adequate pain relief in labour. Non-pharmacological methods are directed at helping prevent the fear of the unknown and perhaps even giving a distraction.

Education of both the mother and her partner is important. This is the role of antenatal classes which may be formal, but even the informal element of meeting other couples is important.

Professional staff who are supportive and well-informed can help decrease anxiety leading to an improvement in pain relief.

Non-pharmacological physical agents include massage, acupuncture and transcutaneous electrical nerve stimulation (TENS). Labouring in water may provide some pain relief. Any of the above would be appropriate answers to Question 1.

Pharmacological agents include:

- Entonox (50% nitrous oxide: 50% oxygen). This is a self-administered agent with very few contraindications. Perhaps the biggest side-effect is that it is commonly used incorrectly and is, therefore, ineffective. Nausea can occur occasionally.

- Pethidine is the narcotic agent most widely used in labour. It has a high instance of side-effects and up to 30% of women experience no relief of pain from it. Side-effects include nausea and vomiting, drowsiness and respiratory depression in the newborn.

Regional analgesia (epidural, spinal) is popular. The latter is usually used only for instrumental deliveries or Caesarean sections.

Contraindications include recent antepartum haemorrhage as well as clotting disorders. Regional analgesias should not be used when there is sepsis at the injection site, active neurological disease, or sensitivity to local analgesia.

Complications associated with regional analgesia include hypotension, respiratory depression, failure to achieve adequate analgesia and a dural puncture leading to headaches.

Recently, chronic backache has been associated with these regional blocks.

Thus, good answers to Question 2 would include:

Pain relief	Contraindication/side-effect
Entonox	ineffective
	nausea
Pethidine	drowsiness
	respiratory distress of the newborn
Epidural	clotting disorder

A pudendal block and other local infiltrations are often used, but they are sometimes ineffective.

Mendelson's syndrome is due to aspiration of gastric contents and is an important contributor to maternal mortality and morbidity.

By increasing the gastric pH to above 3, the syndrome is less likely to occur and that is why histamine-receptor-blocking drugs or alkaline mixtures can help reduce the occurrence of the syndrome.

19

Urinary incontinence is defined by the International Continence Society as an involuntary loss of urine that is objectively shown and a social and hygiene problem. Incontinence can be broadly divided into genuine stress incontinence and an overactive bladder (detrusor instability), other causes include: overflow incontinence, fistula or congenital disorder and urinary tract infection (temporary and the commonest in the elderly). The Key Questions in Evaluating Patients for Urinary Incontinence should include:

- You need to ask about stress incontinence, ie 'Do you leak when you cough, laugh, lift something or sneeze? How often?

- You need to ask about detrusor instability, ie 'Do you have a strong and sudden desire to void (urge) on the way to the bathroom? Do you wet yourself after that? How often?

- Question to identify overflow incontinence, ie Do you ever feel that you are unable to completely empty your bladder?

- Other urinary symptoms like

  How often do you empty your bladder during the day? (Frequency)
  How many times do you get up to urinate after going to sleep? (Nocturia)
  Do you ever leak urine during sex? (Coital incontinence)
  Does it hurt when you urinate? (Dysuria)

The conservative and surgical treatments will depend on the patient's preference, condition and urodynamic diagnosis. Conservative treatment is indicated when patients refuse or are undecided about surgery, they are physically or mentally unfit for surgery or childbearing is incomplete, and there is uncontrolled detrusor instability or voiding difficulty.

Pelvic floor exercises have been successfully used since 1948. The overall rate for cure or much improvement at five years is about 60%. Vaginal cones are useful adjuncts to pelvic floor exercises. A 70% cure or improvement rate was reported after one month's training in cone use. Electrical stimulation for urinary incontinence has been applied with some success by using a variety of appliances at different frequencies. For mild sphincter incompetence, a tampon, reusable foam pessary that supports the bladder neck may temporarily cure incontinence. Also there are several devices which either occlude the urethra or support the bladder neck.

Not all patients with detrusor instability require treatment. Some patients will be able to control their symptoms with simple measures like drinking less, avoiding alcohol, coffee and tea. Conservative methods currently in use to treat detrusor instability are bladder retraining (behavioural intervention), biofeedback, acupuncture, electrical stimulation and anticholinergic drugs.

20

The three forceps shown are:

a. Anderson's non-rotational forceps

b. Kjelland's rotational forceps

c. Wrigley's non-rotational forceps

Forceps can be used in order to speed up delivery and there may be fetal or maternal indications.

Fetal indications include fetal distress and assistance with the after coming head of a breech.

Maternal indications include delay in the second stage and this may include maternal exhaustion. Maternal disease, such as cardiac disease, may be an indication.

It is important that careful assessment of the fetus takes place before delivery and many requirements are satisfied. The requirements include:

- Adequate analgesia, ideally an epidural spinal block.

- The bladder should be empty not only to help decrease bladder injury but also to prevent a full bladder delaying descent of the head.

- It is essential that no obvious cephalopelvic disproportion has been detected. This may be indicated by a large amount of moulding in caput with the head still engaged. It is important, therefore, that the head is not palpable abdominally and is at least 2 cm below the ischial spines.

- The cervix must be fully dilated and the membranes must be ruptured.

- It is important that the position of the head be known and for a non-rotational forceps delivery this should be occipito-anterior.

Any four of the above would be appropriate answers to Question 2.

The second photograph shows a ventouse cup. This can be in metal (as shown) or made of silastic. A ventouse delivery allows a vacuum to be created between the cap and the baby's scalp and then traction is applied to the axis of the birth canal. Indications for use are the same as those for forceps delivery and it is the preferred mode of delivery.

The ventouse has several advantages over the forceps. As it does not occupy any space between the fetal head and the maternal tissue less analgesia may be required. It does appear that there is less risk of maternal and fetal injury. It also allows for fetal rotation to occur and, therefore, if there is any question about the position of the head it would be incorrect to use forceps.

Case
Histories

Case History instructions

The following section contains 10 case history stations in a role-play format so that you can practise your OSCE performance with a colleague.

Choose between you who will play the candidate and who will play the patient, and read the relevant instructions. Throughout the OSCE the person playing the patient should also act as the examiner and mark the candidate accordingly. The answers and mark sheet follows each case history. There are 10 marks to achieve in each station.

STATION 1

Taking a full obstetrics history and antenatal risk assessment

Mrs Khan presents to your antenatal clinic for booking. She is supposed to be 10 weeks pregnant.

Instructions to candidate

1. Obtain a detailed history.

2. Identify any risk factors which may affect her antenatal care.

STATION 1

Taking a full obstetrics history and antenatal risk assessment

Instructions to role player

You are playing the role of Lauer Khan. She is a 39-year-old woman, who is working as a care assistant. It is her fourth pregnancy.

Details of current pregnancy: (2 marks)

- Planned pregnancy with new partner
- LMP: 2/3/03
- Her period is irregular usually every 4–6 weeks, and she bleeds for five days
- She had mild spotting at the beginning of February for couple of days (unusual period)
- Positive pregnancy test at home beginning of April.

Details of previous pregnancies: (2 marks)

- First pregnancy 1995: ended at 10 weeks with missed miscarriage, discovered after having brownish discharge and the pelvic scan. She had ERPC without any complications.
- Second pregnancy 1996: spontaneous vaginal delivery at 39 weeks, healthy boy (David) wt 3.6 kg.
- Third pregnancy 1997: emergency caesarean section at 6 cm dilated for fetal distress, 38 weeks. Healthy girl (Sarah) wt 2.1 kg.

Patient history: (2 marks)

Past gynaecological history:
Last smear test one year ago was normal and always normal.

Past medical history:
Severe from chronic hypertension 1999, on labetalol 200 mg BD.

Past surgical history:
Ruptured appendix 1975, varicose vein procedure in her leg 1998.

Medication:
Labetalol 200 mg BD, iron tablets.

Allergy:
Penicillin.

Smoking:
10 daily (since 1997; during her third pregnancy).

Family history:
Both her parents suffer from hypertension.

Social history:
She is married and lives with her husband and two children

The risk factors in this pregnancy would be: (4 marks)

- Age
- Unreliable LMP (patient was on the pills just two months before the LMP and abnormal spotting)
- Previous caesarean section
- Previous small baby (2.1 kg) + smoking
- Chronic hypertension.

Total marks: 10
Candidate's score:

STATION 2

Communication skills for breaking bad news

Mrs Cunningham, a 58-year-old woman, presents to your surgery with an ultrasound report that shows a large $7 \times 7 \times 6$ cm multi-locular left ovarian cyst with solid components, with a fair amount of free intra-abdominal fluid. Her uterus and other abdominal organs are unremarkable. Mrs Cunningham does not know anything about the scan result. The main objective of this station is to test your skills in doctor–patient communication and breaking bad news, not testing your knowledge in oncology.

Instructions to candidate

Explain to Mrs Cunningham the scan report in a professional manner and take her through the management. You should be able to respond to her concerns.

STATION 2

Communication skills for breaking bad news

Instructions to role player

You are playing the role of Mrs Cunningham who is 58 years old and works as a salesperson. You are very worried and anxious about your health in general and about this scan in particular. You have received an urgent letter from the hospital to see a doctor in one week's time regarding your scan report.

You saw your GP six weeks ago with a history of abdominal distention, bloatedness and bad digestion for the past six months. Your GP performed an abdominal as well as pelvic examination which confirmed a slightly bulky uterus and has meanwhile organised a pelvic ultrasound for you. You haven't seen your GP since.

Patient history:

- P2+0 (2 normal vaginal deliveries 25 and 27 years ago)
- LMP: 6 years ago
- Not on any HRT
- Regular smear test: always normal
- Medically: fit and well
- Past surgical history: not significant
- Non-smoker
- Not on any medication
- No allergies.

Your task:

- Interrupt the candidate and express yourself with tears and anger.
- Insist on having a definite answer as to whether this distention and bloatedness is a cancer or not.
- Be able to evaluate the candidate for his/her counselling skills and manner.

STATION 2

Communication skills for breaking bad news

Marking sheet and suggested answers

Introduction and skills throughout the consultation: (10 marks)

- Introduces self to patient
- Greets patient warmly and with appropriate name
- Maintains good eye contact
- Uses appropriate body posture
- Avoids distracting activities
- Establishes how much the patient knows
- Asks one question at a time
- Explains using language understandable to patient
- Uses silence (allows patient to cry and express anger)
- Shows consideration to the patient's feelings
- Shows understanding, empathy and sensitivity
- Avoids false reassurance (is honest and truthful)
- Listens to concerns
- Makes a plan
- Summarises.

Total marks: 10
Candidate's score:

STATION 3

The menopause

Miss Richter is 51 years old and has come to your clinic with many concerns regarding the menopause. Her last period was roughly 10 months ago and since that time she has developed severe night sweating and hot flushes. She is concerned about the long-term consequences of the menopause and she has made up her mind not to take HRT.

Instructions to candidate

After an appropriate introduction, you have asked Miss Richter if she would like to ask any questions. You should be able to counsel Miss Richter and answer her questions in a professional manner.

STATION 3

The menopause

Instructions to role player

You are playing the role of Miss Richter who is a 51-year-old white woman who had her last period 10 months ago. Your great concern today is regarding osteoporosis and you would like to know whether you are at risk or not and if there are any ways to protect yourself.

Patient profile:

- Caucasian woman
- BMI 18
- Last period 10 months ago
- P0+0
- Smoker: 20 a day for the past 10 years
- Smear always normal
- Normal diet
- Sister had hip fracture at the age of 70 and mother also at the age of 75
- No significant medical Hx
- Not on any HRT and not keen on it.

Remember you are not keen on HRT and your great concern is osteoporosis. You ask the following questions:

1. What are the long-term consequences of the menopause?

2. Am I at risk of osteoporosis?

3. I want to know my risk for osteoporosis. Are there any tests you could offer me?

4. Is there a non-HRT method to protect me from osteoporosis?

5. I am really not keen on HRT. Is there any other treatment for my troublesome hot flushes?

STATION 3

The menopause

Marking sheet and suggested answers

1. **Miss Richter: What are the long-term consequences of the menopause? (2 marks)**

   - Cardiovascular disease: cardiovascular disease is the most common cause of death in women after the age of 60. Coronary heart disease is the commonest cause of death in women in the UK. It is believed that the menopause has adverse effects on the cardiovascular system through the lipoprotein metabolism.

   - Osteoporosis: there is acceleration in bone loss following the menopause; this may result from a decrease in osteoblast activity and an increase in osteoblast activity after the menopause. Fractures of the forearm, hip and vertebrae are the main presentations of osteoporosis.

   - Alzheimer's disease: the incidence of Alzheimer's disease increases significantly after the age of 65. Studies suggest that oestrogen therapy could delay the onset of Alzheimer's disease.

   - Genitourinary atrophy: the vagina and the mucosal lining of the urethra, as well as the trigon of the bladder, appear to undergo atrophic changes after the menopause. As a result postmenopausal women could develop the following symptoms; vaginal dryness, dyspareunia, pruritus, urgency, frequency, dysuria, and incontinence.

2. **Miss Richter: Am I at risk of osteoporosis? (2 marks)**

   To answer this question you should be able to identify and assess the following risk factors by asking the patient specific questions:

   - Underweight (low body mass index)
   - Early menopause (before 45)
   - Corticosteroid therapy
   - Excessive alcohol and caffeine consumption
   - Smoking
   - Low calcium and high protein diet
   - Positive family history (first degree)
   - Chronic diseases (liver, hyperparathyroidism, hyperthyroidism)
   - Caucasian origin
   - Nulliparity.

3. Miss Richter: I want to know my risk for osteoporosis. Is there any test you could offer me? (2 marks)

Obviously Miss Richter is at high risk to develop osteoporosis. There are two main tests:

1. DEXA (dual energy X-ray absorptiometry): this test measures the bone mineral density (BMD) usually at the spine and the hip.

2. Ultrasound can be used to measure bone structure in the heel or in the shin.

4. Miss Richter: What about osteoporosis, is there a non-HRT method to protect me from it? (2 marks)

A good answer should include:

-   Eat a balanced diet
-   Stop smoking
-   Limit alcohol intake
-   Regular exercise
-   Calcium and vitamin D 1000–1500 mg of calcium supplements a day.

5. Miss Richter: I am really not keen on HRT. Is there any other treatment for my troublesome hot flushes? (2 marks)

Patient wishes and decisions should always be respected. A good answer should explore all the treatment options for hot flushes.

-   The most effective treatment for hot flushes caused by the menopause is oestrogens; however recent studies show that oestrogens given after the menopause increases a woman's risk for breast cancer, heart attacks and strokes
-   Treatment with progestogen, such as megestrol acetate (40 mg/day) or norethisterone 5 mg/day can reduce the frequency and severity of hot flushes
-   Oral clonidine
-   A high intake of dietary phyto-oestrogens
-   Vitamin E
-   Selective serotonin-reuptake inhibitors such as venlafaxine
-   Exercise and change in life style.

Total marks: 10
Candidate's score:

STATION 4

Amniocentesis counselling

Mrs Wood is 41 years old with her first pregnancy. She has made an appointment to see you at 10 weeks' gestation with a list of questions regarding amniocentesis and Down's syndrome.

Instructions to candidate

1. After an appropriate introduction, you have asked Mrs Wood if she would like to ask any questions.

2. You should be able to counsel Mrs Wood and answer her questions in a professional manner.

STATION 4

Amniocentesis counselling

Instructions to role player

You are playing the role of Mrs Wood who is a 41-year-old lawyer with her first pregnancy. Her partner is a 49-year-old schoolteacher. She feels very happy being pregnant but she feels that she can't cope with a child with Down's syndrome. Her sister had a child with Down's syndrome at the age of 32. You should be able to initiate a conversation about your worries of having a child with Down's syndrome. You should be willing to explore all of the available diagnostic options in detail.

You should explore the following

1. What is the risk of me having a baby with Down's syndrome?

2. Does my partner's age increases my risk?

3. When is the best time to perform the amniocentesis?

4. What information can you tell me about early amniocentesis and its safety?

5. Is the procedure painful?

6. What are the complications?

7. When will the result be available?

8. Can this result guarantee a normal healthy baby?

STATION 4

Amniocentesis counselling

Marking and answer sheet

1. Risk of Down's syndrome at age 40: (1 mark)

Down's syndrome (trisomy 21) is the commonest cause of mental retardation. The prevalence of Down's syndrome increases with maternal age. The risk increases from 1:1000 at age 30 to 1:100 at age 40.

2. Partner's age: (1 mark)

The partner's age adds no risk to the incidence of Down's syndrome.

3. Timing of amniocentesis: (1 mark)

Although early amniocentesis is possible, the usual timing for amniocentesis is between 14 and 16 weeks of pregnancy.

4. Early amniocentesis and its safety: (1 mark)

Early amniocentesis before 14 weeks is possible and the technique is similar to that performed at 14 to 16 weeks. However, early amniocentesis (before 14 weeks) appears to be associated with significant problems, including increased fetal loss rate, fetal talipes and a reduced amniocyte culture rate compared to those procedures performed at 15 weeks.

5. Is the procedure painful? (1 mark)

The procedure should not be painful but may be associated with some discomfort and mild abdominal cramp afterwards.

6. Possible complications: (3 marks)

The main complication associated with amniocentesis is the risk of miscarriage and this risk has been estimated to be 0.5–1%. Most of these occur in the first three to four weeks following the procedure. There is a 2–3% risk of rhesus iso-immunisation following amniocentesis due to feto-maternal haemorrhage therefore anti-D should be given to all rhesus negative women at the time of the test. Vaginal bleeding, abdominal pain and leaking of amniotic fluid have been reported within 72 hours of amniocentesis in more than 3% of women. Congenital hip dislocation, talipes, equinovarus and low birth weight occur more often after amniocentesis, and neonatal respiratory difficulties have been reported to be significantly high in babies born to women who had an amniocentesis during the pregnancy. Finally, amniocentesis can be associated with culture failure especially when the amniotic fluid is contaminated by blood.

7. Availability of the results: (2 marks)

The aim of amniocentesis is to obtain tissue of the same genetic origin as the fetus and use these cells for chromosomal analysis. Because of the difficulties in using uncultured cells, the amniotic cells are usually cultured for two weeks then used for testing for chromosomal abnormalities, and metabolic and biochemical disorders. The client should be forewarned she may not receive the results for up to 14 days. On the other hand, other methods rather than karyotyping have been used to examine the amniotic fluid cells for chromosomal abnormalities in pregnancy. These techniques are based on DNA analysis of uncultured cells (PCR and FISH) and the results are usually available in a couple of days.

8. Can this negative result guarantee a normal healthy baby? (1 mark)

No prenatal test can guarantee the birth of a healthy baby. There is always a risk of laboratory and technical error as well as false positive and false negative results. The failure rate of amniocentesis averages at 0.4%. Amniocentesis cannot exclude structural congenital abnormalities and birth defects.

Total marks: 10
Candidate's score:

STATION 5

Emergency contraception

You are on call in a busy obstetric unit and you have been asked to see a very stressed 20-year-old woman who has had unprotected intercourse and is seeking your advice regarding emergency contraception.

Instructions to candidate

Deal with this woman, take a brief history and counsel her regarding emergency contraception, answering all her concerns.

STATION 5

Emergency contraception

Instructions to role player

You are a very stressed university student who had unprotected inter-course last night (less than 24 hours ago). You have never used emergency contraception and your knowledge regarding contraception in general is limited.

Patient profile:

- 21 years old
- P0+1 (previous TOP three years ago, uncomplicated)
- Not in a established relationship and not using contraception at the moment
- LMP = 12 days ago; period is regular and every 28 days and bleed for five days
- Medically you are fit and well and no previous surgeries however had a previous episode of pelvic inflammatory disease, which was treated with IV antibiotics at hospital two years ago
- No allergies
- Smokes socially
- Drink only at weekends
- Live with three other students in a flat
- No medication.

Your task:

You are shy and stressed about having unprotected sex. You are not ready to have a baby so your aim is to explore in detail the options available, their side effects and success rates. You should ask the following questions:

1. How many types of emergency contraception are available and what would you offer me?

2. How do I take these pills? (Only ask if the candidate offers you emergency pills)

3. How effective is the emergency pill? (Only ask if the candidate offers you emergency pills)

4. What happens if I have intercourse after taking the pills?

5. What are the side effects of the emergency pill?

6. When should my next period come?

STATION 5

Emergency contraception

Marking sheet and suggested answers

Introduction: (2 marks)

- Introduces self to patient
- Greets patient warmly
- Maintains good eye contact
- Uses appropriate body posture
- Asks one question at a time
- Explains using language understandable to patient
- Listens to concerns
- Summarises.

History taking: (2 marks)

A good history should include:

- The time of the intercourse
- The last menstrual periods
- The type of contraception used if any
- Any serious medical conditions
- Establishing if she has used this type of pill before
- Her previous obstetrics history.

Counselling the patient: (6 marks)

1. How many types of emergency contraception are available and what would you offer me?
There are three main types of emergency contraception:

- Combined hormonal method (PC4, Ovran)
- Progestogen-only emergency contraception (levonorgestrel method)
- Insertion of a copper IUD.

This patient is a good candidate for progestogen-only emergency contraception as it is proved to be more effective and has fewer side effects than the combined method. This patient is not a good candidate for the IUCD as she had intercourse less than 24 hours ago and has no children.

2. How do I take these pills? (Only ask if the candidate offers you emergency pills)

The patient should swallow the first tablet as soon as possible (it should be within 72 hours of the unprotected intercourse), followed by a second tablet 12 hours later. If taking the second dose 12 hours later would be difficult, the timing of the second dose might be altered to suit social hours. The patient should be advised to repeat the dose if she vomits within two hours of taking the tablet.

3. How effective is the emergency pill? (Only ask if the candidate offers you emergency pills)

The progestogen-only emergency contraception method will prevent 89% of conceptions.

4. What happens if I have intercourse after taking the pills?

Emergency contraceptive pills will not protect against pregnancy from intercourse that occurs after the pills are taken.

5. What are the side effects of the emergency pill?

There are no long-term or serious side effects. Almost all women can safely use this emergency pill. Some women may experience vomiting or may feel sick.

6. When should my next period come?

Next period is unpredictable. Period can come on time, earlier, later or some women could have irregular bleeding. The most important thing that the patient should be aware of is the risk of pregnancy and a pregnancy test should be performed if the period is delayed by three weeks.

Total marks: 10
Candidate's score:

STATION 6

Urinary incontinence

Mrs Robinson, a 59-year-old woman, presents to your surgery with history of urinary incontinence for the last five months.

Instructions to candidate

1. Obtain a detailed history and examination.

2. Name four tests which may be helpful for diagnosis.

STATION 6

Urinary incontinence

Instructions to role player
You are playing Mrs Robinson. You should present this case in a sensible and logical manner.

Patient profile:
Mrs Robinson is 59 years old; she works in a charity shop. Her current problem: is leaking a small amount of urine when she coughs or sneezes and when lifting heavy objects. This problem started eight months ago and has gradually increased in the last five months with several embarrassing occasions at work. She feels that her social life has been slightly affected by this problem.

Other urinary symptoms:
She passes a good amount of urine between five and eight times a day (no frequency) and wakes up once at night (no nocturia). She has no difficulty or pain when passing urine (dysuria). Occasionally she has a strong desire to pass urine (urgency) and on very few occasions (three times in the last five months) has wet herself following the urgency feeling (urge incontinence). She has never wet herself whilst sleeping (no nocturnal enuresis). Mrs Robinson is not sexually active (no coital incontinence). She is not aware of any other gynaecological problems (no vaginal discharge and no vaginal prolapse). Her fluid intake including caffeine is normal.

LMP: 5 years ago. She is not on HRT.

Para 3+1:
Three previous normal vaginal births 25, 23 and 20 years ago. Birth weights 3.5 kg, 3.8 kg and 4.2 kg respectively. A miscarriage at eight weeks' gestation 30 years ago, no complications.

Past gynaecological history:
Last cervical smear one year ago, normal. Mrs Robinson has one abnormal cervical smear 15 years ago for which she had laser treatment (LLETZ) followed by normal smears to date. No other significant gynaecological problems.

Past medical history:
She suffers from long-term depression and she is currently on medication.

Past surgical history:
Appendectomy 40 years ago. Left ovarian cystectomy 19 years ago.

Medication:
Antidepressant (Prozac).

Allergies:
Penicillin.

Smoking:
10 a day for 20 years.

Social life:
Mrs Robinson lives with her husband who suffered a car accident five years ago resulting in disability. She is very active and enjoys walking and swimming.

On examination:
(only if candidate asks for examination results.) Mrs Robinson is fit and well, BMI 23.

Abdominal examination:
Soft, lax, not tender, there was a large suprapubic mass. Bikini line incision and appendix scar noticed.

Speculum examination:
No abnormalities detected. No urinary incontinence during examination or when patient asked to cough.

Bimanual examination:
16-week size uterus, mobile, not tender and both adnexa free.

STATION 6

Urinary incontinence

Marking sheet and suggested answers
Introduction and communication skills: (3 marks)

- Makes appropriate introduction
- Greets patient warmly and with appropriate name
- Maintain eye to eye contact
- Asks one question at a time
- Explains using language understandable to patient
- Shows understanding, empathy and sensitivity
- Listens to concerns
- Summarises
- Evaluates patient.

History taking: (3 marks)
A good candidate should explore the following:

- Current problem and duration
- Other urinary symptoms such as: frequency, nocturia, dysuria, urgency, urge incontinence, nocturnal enuresis and coital incontinence
- Other gynaecological problems (vaginal discharge and vaginal prolapse)
- LMP+ HRT
- Parity and mode of delivery
- Past gynaecological history
- Past medical history
- Past surgical history
- Medication
- Allergies
- Smoking
- Social life.

The following tests may be helpful: (4 marks)

- Midstream urine specimen for culture and sensitivity
- Frequency volume chart (volume voided chart)
- Pad test (simple, non-invasive test to detect urinary leaking)
- Urodynamic study
- Pelvic ultrasound to identify the size and nature of the pelvic mass.

Total marks: 10
Candidate's score:

STATION 7

Menorrhagia

Mrs Pearson is 42 years old. She has heavy regular periods. She has come to your clinic for the second time to discuss the results of her diagnostic hysteroscopy and endometrial biopsy, which was performed four weeks ago.

Instructions to candidate

Explain to Mrs Pearson the operative findings and the pros and cons of each treatment option. Refer to the history sheet, operative notes and histopathology result when discussing her results.

General Hospital

NAME: Mrs Pearson

PATIENT ID NO: D345678

DOB: 03/12/1960

HISTORY SHEET

06/08/03

P2+1

2 caesarean sections

LMP: 2 weeks ago

Contraception: vasectomy

Smear: regular/up-dated/always normal

C/O: Heavy regular periods for 6 years.
   Flooding with large clots
   Bleed for 7 days all heavy every 28 days
   Had anaemia and blood transfusion
   No PCB
   No IMB
   No dysmenorrhoea

Past medical history: non-significant.
Past surgical history: two previous caesarean sections and previous
laparotomy and left salpingectomy for left ectopic pregnancy 15 years ago.
Not on any medication and no allergies
Doesn't smoke, and lives with her husband happily.

On examination:

Looks well and fit

Abdominal Ex: soft, lax, no masses

Speculum: Normal looking cervix
            No abnormal vaginal discharge seen

VE/   NS/AV/mobile uterus
        adnexa free

P/   patient anxious would like to proceed to hysteroscopy and
        endometrial biopsy

Booked for HEB/biopsy

General Hospital
Department of Histology and Cytology

NAME: Mrs Pearson
DOB: 03/12/1960
AGE/SEX: 42Y F

PATIENT ID NO: D345678
LAB NO: DR-5678

CONULTANT/GP: Mr Smith
LOCATION: Theatre 5

Specimen date: 06/09/2003
Specimen time: 1420

SPECIMEN(S)
Endometrial, biopsy

CLINICAL DETAILS
Menorrhagia

MACRO
Brown tissue fragment all embedded in one block.

MICRO
Secretory endometrium with tissue representation also from the lower uterine segment. No evidence of malignancy.

DR K. L. M. N.

General Hospital
Day Surgery Unit

Operative Notes

DATE: 06/09/2003
SURGEON: Mr Jones
PROCEDURE: Hysteroscopy & Endometrial biopsy

EUA: NS/AV/mobile uterus
        adnexa free

uncomplicated hysteroscopy
clear view
both ostia seen
no intra-uterine abnormalities
thin endometrium

endometrial biopsy ---------------- tissue +++ -------------- (H)

GOP 4 WEEKS

HOME TONIGHT

STATION 7

Menorrhagia

Instructions to role player

This problem is causing you a great amount of stress so you feel very determined to explore all of your treatment options in detail with your doctor. Your aim is to discuss each treatment option, its effectiveness, side effects and its suitability for you. You should keep asking: are there any more options?

You have heard about the 'ten-minute hysterectomy' and you are interested in finding out more.

Summary of patient profile:

You are 42 years old, working as a teacher in the local high school. You have two grown up children who are 20 and 18 years old, both delivered by emergency caesarean section for fetal distress.

Your current problem started six years ago when you decided to stop the combined contraception pill after your husband had a vasectomy. You have a heavy regular period every 28 days and you bleed for seven days with clots. This has caused many embarrassing occasions at school and as a result of your heavy periods you have been admitted to the hospital with anaemia and you have had a blood transfusion just five weeks ago.

- You are still complaining of heavy periods and your LMP was two weeks ago.
- You have regular cervical smear which has always been normal.
- Past medical history: non-significant.
- Past surgical history: two previous caesarean sections and previous laparotomy and left salpingectomy for left ectopic pregnancy 15 years ago.
- Not on any medication and no allergies
- You don't smoke and you live with your husband happily.

STATION 7

Menorrhagia

Marking sheet and suggested answers

Introduction and explanation skills: (4 marks)

- Introduces self to patient
- Greets patient
- Maintains good eye contact
- Explains using language understandable to patient (avoiding medical jargon)
- Asks one question at a time
- Uses balanced counselling
- Listens to concerns and asks if patient wants to ask any more questions
- Summarises and asks if the patient fully understood.

Treatment options: (6 marks)

Both medical and surgical treatments have side effects. A good candidate should explore the following treatment options:

1. Antifibrinolytic drugs

- Methods of use
- Effectiveness
- Side effects.

Antifibrinolytic drugs (tranexamic acid) and prostaglandin synthetase inhibitors (mefenamic acid) cause 50% reduction in the blood loss. They should be given only during menstruation. Side effects of tranexamic acid include: nausea, vomiting, diarrhoea, and disturbances in colour vision and rarely thromboembolic events. It is usually considered as a first-line treatment option. Mefenamic acid has minor anti-inflammatory properties. Occasionally, it can cause diarrhoea and haemolytic anaemia.

2. Prostaglandin synthetase inhibitors

- Methods of use
- Effectiveness
- Side effects.

3. Progestogen therapy

Oral route

- Method of use
- Effectiveness
- Side effects.

Therapy with oral progestins results in a 15% to 25% reduction in menstrual blood flow when used alone. Common side effects include moodiness, breakthrough bleeding, weight gain, headaches, and breast tenderness. They can be given for 10–14 days during the luteal phase.

Intramuscular route

- Method of use
- Effectiveness
- Side effects.

Progestins can be given intramuscularly as a form of Depo Provera injection and this can cause irregular withdrawal bleeding. The majority of women will have amenorrhoea within a year.

Danazol
- Side effects
- Suitability for this patient in a long-term use.

Combined contraceptive pill
- Other benefits
- Suitability for this patient.

4. Mirena coil

- Effectiveness
- Suitability
- Side effects.

This IUCD contains progestins, which are released locally and mainly affect the uterus and the cervix. As a result it has fewer side effects than the oral or intramuscular routes. Irregular break-through bleeding can occur for the first three to six months. Mirena coil provides an effective treatment for menorrhagia (80% to 90% reduction in blood loss within six months) and is also an effective and reversible form of contraception.

5. Minimum invasive surgery

- Awareness of old methods
- Second generation and their effectiveness
- Issues related to long-term outcome like amenorrhoea, pregnancy, endometrial cancer and Combined HRT.

Minimal access treatments for menorrhagia include first generation techniques such as transcervical resection of endometrium (TCRE) and rollerball ablation. The second generation techniques include balloon thermal ablation.

6. Hysterectomy
Morbidity and mortality of this surgery.

Hysterectomy: hysterectomy provides a definitive cure for menorrhagia, but is associated with substantial postoperative recovery time and morbidity. The mortality associated with hysterectomy depends on several factors such as age, surgical approach and associated conditions and it varies from 0.1 to 1 in 1000 procedures.

Balloon thermal ablation: recent studies report a high satisfaction rate of up to 85%, however long-term studies are awaited. This procedure is performed under general anaesthesia AS A DAY-CASE. Postoperative morbidity, hospital stay, and recovery time are significantly less after endometrial ablation than after hysterectomy.

Total marks: 10
Candidate's score

STATION 8

Interactive with the examiner

Interact with the examiner by answering the following questions.

Instructions to candidate

You have been asked to see a woman aged 26 years at casualty with lower abdominal pain and mild vaginal bleeding. Her LMP was seven weeks ago and she does not use any contraception. Medically and surgically she is fit and well.

STATION 8

Interactive with the examiner

Instructions to role player

You are playing the role of the examiner. Ask the following questions:

1. Give me four differential diagnoses

2. Let us assume it is miscarriage. So, how many types of miscarriages are there?

3. How would you differentiate between threatened miscarriage and inevitable miscarriage?

4. What is the incidence of ectopic pregnancy?

5. What is the most common site for ectopic pregnancy?

6. Give five risk factors for ectopic pregnancy

7. What are the surgical options to treat ectopic pregnancy?

8. Is there any medical treatment for ectopic pregnancy?

STATION 8

Interactive with the examiner

Marking sheet and suggested answers

1. Examiner: Give me four differential diagnoses. (1 mark)

A good answer should include:

- Miscarriage
- Ectopic pregnancy
- Molar pregnancy
- Delayed period with dysmenorrhoea.

2. Examiner: Let us assume it is miscarriage. So, how many types of miscarriages are there? (1 mark)

- **Threatened miscarriage:** light bleeding +/– mild Abd pain and a closed cervix; 50% of the cases settle down
- **Inevitable miscarriage:** heavy bleeding (clots) + severe Abd pain and the cervix is usually open
- **Incomplete miscarriage:** same as above + has passed part of the product (tissues, placenta or membranes)
- **Complete miscarriage:** spontaneous expulsion of all products + ↓ bleeding and pain and usually cervix closed
- **Delayed or missed miscarriage:** early symptoms of pregnancy subside +/– bleeding (usually by chance by scan)
- **Septic miscarriage:** pyrexia, discharge.
- **Recurrent miscarriage**

3. Examiner: How would you differentiate between threatened miscarriage and inevitable miscarriage? (1 mark)

History and clinical examination are important. From the history the threatened miscarriage usually associates with mild bleeding (spotting) as well as a mild abdominal pain. On examination the cervix is usually closed, and the vaginal bleeding minimum. However, the inevitable miscarriage will associate with heavy vaginal bleeding with clots sometimes and severe abdominal pain. On examination it is not uncommon to see a dilated cervix with product passing through it.

4. Examiner: What is the incidence of ectopic pregnancy? (1 mark)

Incidence of ectopic pregnancy has increased over the last few decades. It is estimated that 1 in 80 to 1 in 120 of all pregnancies is ectopic. The risk of recurrence is 10–20%.

5. Examiner: What is the most common site for ectopic pregnancy? (2 marks)

97% of ectopic pregnancies are tubal and the ampulla is the most common tubal site of implantation.

6. Examiner: Give five risk factors for ectopic pregnancy. (1 mark)

Remember that 45% of all ectopic pregnancies have no risk factors. However the following factors increase the likehood of ectopic pregnancy:

- PID (6–10 times higher than in women with no previous history of PID)
- Tubal surgery (20% after sterilization)
- IVF treatment (2–5% of clinical pregnancies are ectopic with IVF)
- Previous ectopic pregnancy and previous surgery for ectopic pregnancy
- IUCD and progesterone-only contraception
- Smoking
- Tubal anomalies.

7. Examiner: What are the surgical options to treat ectopic pregnancy? (1 mark)

There are two surgical approaches to treat ectopic pregnancy. First, is the laparoscopic approach. The major advantages of this approach are quick recovery, less hospital stay and less pain. However this approach is not suitable for a shocked patient or in patient with large intra-abdominal bleed. The second approach is laparotomy.

The following procedures can be done to treat ectopic pregnancy:

- Salpingotomy (or -ostomy): making an incision on the tube and removing the pregnancy
- Salpingectomy: taking the tube out
- Segmental resection: taking out the affected portion of the tube.

8. **Examiner: Is there any medical treatment for ectopic pregnancy? (2 marks)**

The first ectopic pregnancy to be treated medically was in 1985. Good results with very few side effects are seen with use of methotrexate, a single intramuscular dose of 50 mg.

Selection criteria for methotrexate:

- Hemodynamically stable
- No evidence of tubal rupture or significant intra-abdominal haemorrhage
- The ectopic pregnancy is less than 3–4 cm in diameter
- No contraindications to MTX
- Patient will be available for protracted follow-up.

Total marks: 10
Candidate's score:

STATION 9

Interactive with the examiner

Interact with the examiner by answering the following questions.

Instructions to candidate

A 23-year-old woman presents to the Emergency Department with severe lower abdominal pain for the last 10 hours, foul vaginal discharge for three days, with vomiting and nausea. Her LMP was five days ago and she has used the combined contraceptive pill for the last five years.

STATION 9

Interactive with the examiner

Instructions to role player

You are playing the role of the examiner. Ask the following questions:

1. Give four differential diagnoses for this case.

2. Give five risk factors for pelvic inflammatory disease.

3. Name five important clinical findings to support your diagnosis of acute PID.

4. What are the long-term consequences of acute PID?

5. What is the value of pelvic ultrasound in diagnosis of acute PID?

6. When would you refer a patient with PID for hospital based treatment? Give four referral criteria.

7. What follow-up and what advice would you give after three days of successful hospital based treatment for acute PID?

STATION 9

Interactive with the examiner

Marking sheet and suggested answers

1. Examiner: Give four differential diagnoses for this case. (1 mark)

A good answer should include the following:

- Pelvic inflammatory disease
- Surgical emergencies (appendicitis)
- Ectopic pregnancy
- Ovarian pathology (torsion, rupture).

2. Examiner: Give five risk factors for pelvic inflammatory disease. (2 marks)

A good answer should include the following:

- Age and especially young age at first intercourse (adolescents are three times more at risk than women who are 25–30 years old)
- Multiple sexual partners
- IUCD (high risk of PID occurs during the first 20 days)
- Smoking
- Vaginal douching
- Combined contraceptive pills.

3. Examiner: Name five important clinical findings to support your diagnosis of acute PID (2 marks)

A good answer should include the following:

- Lower abdominal tenderness on palpation
- Bilateral adnexal tenderness on vaginal examination
- Cervical excitation on vaginal examination
- Oral temperature more than 38°C
- Abnormal cervical or vaginal discharge
- Elevated WBC (more than 10,000)
- Elevated C-reactive protein.

4. Examiner: What are the long-term consequences of acute PID? (1 mark)

A good answer should include:

- Ectopic pregnancy is six to seven times more likely to occur in women who have had PID compared with a control group.
- Tubal damage and scarring can result in infertility. One study demonstrated infertility in 40% of women after three or more episodes.
- Chronic pelvic pain in up to 18% of women after PID had resolved. This can lead to frequent hospitalisation, and hysterectomy rates are 10 times higher.

5. Examiner: What is the value of pelvic ultrasound in diagnosis of acute PID? (1 mark)

Pelvic ultrasound is not used in the routine diagnosis of uncomplicated PID, however it is a valuable in the diagnosis of tubo-ovarian abscess and ovarian cyst.

6. Examiner: When would you refer a patient with PID for hospital based treatment? Give four referral criteria. (2 marks)

A good answer should include the following:

- When the surgical emergencies cannot be excluded
- The patient is not responding to oral antibiotics
- The patient is unable to tolerate an outpatient oral regimen
- Acute episodes (severe abdominal pain and high fever)
- Suspected tubo-ovarian abscess
- The patient is immunodeficient.

7. Examiner: What follow up and what advice would you give after three days of successful hospital based treatment for acute PID? (1 mark)

- Advise to continue oral antibiotics for a full two weeks
- Advise that treatment of sexual contacts is essential to prevent re-infection
- Advise follow-up visit at clinic for swabs
- Advise regarding safe sex and how to prevent further attacks
- Advise about future pregnancies and possibility of ectopic pregnancy.

Total marks: 10
Candidate's score:

STATION 10

Interactive with the examiner

Interact with the examiner by answering the following questions.

Instructions to candidate

Miss Woodfin had an emergency caesarean section for severe fetal distress in labour at 5 cm dilatation. Miss Woodfin is 39 years old and was in her first pregnancy.

STATION 10

Interactive with the examiner

Instructions to role player

You are playing the role of the examiner. Ask the candidate to respond to the following:

1. Four hours after Miss Woodfin's caesarean section, you are asked by midwives whether Miss Woodfin will need prophylactic anticoagulant. How would you decide?

2. Next morning, you are asked to assess and perform a post-caesarean section check-up. Take the examiner through a routine postnatal examination. You will be asked to justify each step in your examination.

3. Three days later, Miss Woodfin complains of high fever; her temperature in two consecutive reading (four hours apart) is 38°C. List five possible causes for her fever with their appropriate investigations.

STATION 10

Interactive with the examiner

Marking sheet and suggested answers

1. Four hours after Miss Woodfin's caesarean section, you are asked by midwives whether Miss Woodfin needs prophylactic anticoagulant. How would you decide? (3 marks)

Pulmonary thromboembolism (PTE) remains the main cause of maternal death in the UK. A good answer to this question should include a full review of Miss Woodfin's antenatal notes and her past medical and surgical history, as well as her general health and appearance, looking for certain risk factors which increase the likelihood for postnatal thrombosis. These risk factors related to the postnatal period include the following:

- Emergency caesarean section
- Age > 35
- Obesity
- Previous history of DVT
- Heart diseases
- Prolonged bed rest (paralysis/ fractures).

Most obstetricians would commence anticoagulant therapy after an emergency caesarean section in presence of any other risk factor.

2. Next morning, you are asked to assess and perform a post-caesarean section check-up. Take the examiner through a routine postnatal examination. You will be asked to justify each step in your examination. (3 marks)

- General appearance (orientation, dehydration, pain, posture.)
- Vital signs (BP, pulse, temperature)
- Examine the eyes looking for jaundice or anaemia
- Listen to the chest and examine the breast if there is specific complaint
- Examine the abdomen and the fundal height and listen to the bowel
- Feel gently the wound to be sure there is no haematoma and it is not oozing
- Examine the legs looking for DVT
- Review the catheter (including input and output).

Also you would be expected to ask about the following:

- Breast feeding
- Pain
- Bleeding (lochia)
- Respiratory symptoms
- Urinary or bowel symptoms
- Mood swinging and sleeping.

3. Three days later, Miss Woodfin complains of high fever; her temperature in two consecutive reading (four hours apart) is 38°C. List five possible causes for her fever with their appropriate investigations. (4 marks)

The most common cause for puerperal pyrexia is endometritis (an infection of the endometrium or decidua, with extension into the myometrium and parametrial tissues). Endometritis is a polymicrobial infection involving both aerobic and anaerobic organisms that commonly occurs in the first seven days after delivery. Other causes for puerperal pyrexia would includes: wound infection, wound haematoma, pelvic cellulitis, cystitis, pyelonephritis, breast engorgement, mastitis, pneumonia and septic pelvic thrombophlebitis.

The diagnosis of endometritis is based on clinical findings including fever, lower abdominal pain, uterine tenderness, and foul-smelling lochia. The abdominal wound should be carefully evaluated for signs of infection. A rectovaginal examination should be done to rule out parametritis or any pelvic abscess and haematoma. A complete blood count, urinalysis, urine culture, blood culture and vaginal swabs should be performed. An abdominal CT scan would be indicated in a patient who fails to respond to adequate antimicrobial therapy.

Total Marks: 10
Candidate's score:

Recommended Reading List

Books available from the RCOG Bookshop:
27 Sussex Place, Regent's Park, London, NW1 4RG
www.rcog.org.uk/bookshop

Anthony, J, Kaye P, *Notes for the DRCOG, 4th Edition* (London: Churchill Livingstone, 2001)

Benrubi, G I, *Handbook of Obstetric and Gynaecologic Emergencies* (Philadelphia: J B Lippincott, 2001)

Boue, A, *Fetal Medicine: Prenatal Diagnosis and Management* (Oxford: Oxford University Press, 1995)

Campbell, S, Lees, C, *Obstetrics by Ten Teachers, 17th Edition* (London: Arnold, 2000)

Chamberlain, G, Bowen-Simpkins, P, *A Practice of Obstetrics and Gynaecology: A Textbook for General Practice and the DRCOG, Third Edition* (London: Churchill Livingstone, 2000)

Chamberlain, G, *Turnbull's Obstetrics, 3rd Edition* (London: Churchill Livingstone, 2001)

Campbell, S, Monga, A, *Gynaecology by Ten Teachers, 17th Edition* (London: Arnold, 2000)

Chamberlain, G W, Hamilton-Fairley, D, *Lecture Notes on Obstetrics and Gynaecology* (London: Blackwell, 1999)

Chamberlain, G, Morgan, M, *ABC of Antenatal Care, 4th Edition* (London: BMJ Books, 2002)

Coales, U, *DRCOG: MCQs and OSCEs – How to pass first time* (London: RSM Press, 2002)

Green Top Guidelines, *Royal College of Obstetricians and Gynaecologists*

Guillebaud, J, *Contraception: Your Questions Answered, 4th Edition* (London: Churchill Livingstone, 2003)

Gupta, J K, Mires, G, Khan, K S, *Core Clinical Cases and Obstetrics and Gynaecology* – a problem solving approach (London: Arnold, 2001)

Hoghton, M, Hogston, P, *MCQs for the DRCOG, 2nd Edition* (London: Churchill Livingstone, 1999)

James, D, Steer, P, Weiner, C, Gonik, B, *High-risk pregnancy management options, 2nd Edition* (London: Saunders, 1999)

James, D K, Johnson, I R, McEwan, A, *An Obstetrics and Gynaecology Vade-Mecum* (London: Arnold, 2000)

Llewllyn-Jones, D, *Fundamentals of Obstetrics and Gynaecology, 7th Edition* (London: Mosby, 1999)

McCormack, M J, Duthie, S J, Khaled, M A, *The Complete DRCOG – OSCEs, MCQs, Revision Notes* (London: Saunders, 2001)

Rees, M, Pudie, D W, *Management of the Menopause* (London: BMS Publications, 2002)

Rymer, J, Ahmed, H, *OSCEs in Obstetrics and Gynaecology* (London: Churchill Livingstone, 1998)

Rymer, J, Davis, G, Rodin, A and Chapman, M, *Preparation and Revision for the DRCOG, 3rd Edition,* (London: Churchill Livingstone, 2003)

Rymer, J, Higham, J, *Preparing for the DRCOG: MCQs and Case Studies* (London: Petroc Press, 1994)

Setchell, M, Thilagananthan, B, *Ten Teachers' Self-Assessment in Gynaecology and Obstetrics – Multiple Choice and Short Answer Questions* (London: Arnold, 2001)

Shaw, R W, Soutter, W P, and Stanton, S L, *Gynaecology, 3rd Edition* (London: Churchill Livingstone, 2002)

de Swiet, M, Chamberlain, G, Bennett, P, *Basic Science in Obstetrics and Gynaecology* (London: Churchill Livingstone, 2001)

Ward, N, Leck I, *Antenatal and neonatal screening, 2nd Edition* (Oxford: Oxford University Press, 2000)

Whitehead, M, Godfree, V, *HRT Your Questions Answered, 2nd Edition* (Churchill Livingstone, 1996)

Why Mothers Die 1997–1999 'Report on Confidential Enquiry into Maternal Deaths in the United Kingdom'. HMSO

Index

PASTEST DRCOG INTENSIVE REVISION COURSES

With over 30 years of experience in postgraduate medical education, PasTest offers DRCOG candidates an intensive revision course which provides the practice you need to succeed.

Courses

We run courses for both Diploma Examination sittings at our centres in London and Manchester. Our four day courses provide comprehensive preparation for both the MCQ and OSCE elements of the examination. Subject-based lectures will guide you through all aspects of the syllabus including Menopause and HRT, Subfertility and Primary Care and Neonatology. During the four days you will complete two 22 station OSCE circuits including interactive stations designed to improve your factual knowledge, problem solving, diagnosis, investigation and treatment and communication skills.

The course features:

- Comprehensive course material, including over 200 MCQs
- Pre-course examination to identify areas of weakness
- Skilled tutors with many years' DRCOG teaching experience
- Realistic OSCE circuits for essential examination experience

The course focuses on key topics for the DRCOG, including menstrual disorders, abnormal cervical smear, urology, maternal infection, contraception, infertility, neonatal problems and sexually transmitted diseases.

PasTest's teaching material is designed to help busy exam candidates use their revision time effectively, by concentrating on the questions and answers that really count. We are proud of our high pass rate.
Contact PasTest today for full details:

PasTest, Freepost, Egerton Court, Parkgate Estate, Knutsford, Cheshire, WA16 7BR
Tel: 01565 752000 Fax: 01565 650264 Website: www.pastest.co.uk